Teaching and Learning Nursing Ethics

Edited by

Ursula Gallagher BSc (Hons) RGN
K M Boyd MA BD PhD

Scutari Press

A division of Scutari Projects, the publishing company of
the Royal College of Nursing

First published 1991

British Library Cataloguing in Publication Data
Teaching and learning nursing ethics.
   1. Medicine. Nursing. Ethical aspects
   I. Gallagher, Ursula II. Boyd, Kenneth M.
   174.2

   ISBN 1-871364-38-8

Typeset by MC Typeset Ltd., Gillingham, Kent
Printed and bound in Great Britain by Billing & Sons, Worcester

Teaching and Learning Nursing Ethics

Contents

The Working Party

Professor Jenifer Wilson-Barnett (Chairman)
RGN DipN BA MSc PhD RNT FRCN
Dept of Nursing Studies
King's College
London

The Pilot Group
Miss Mary Armstrong BA RGN
The Revd Kenneth Boyd MA BD PhD (Research Fellow)
Miss Sylvia P Docking MA RGN RM RNT
Mrs Maureen Macmillan BA PhD RGN
Prebendary E F Shotter BA
Mr Richard Rowson BA (Visiting Fellow)
Ms Ursula Gallagher BSc RGN (Research Assistant)

The Working Party
Miss Pat Ashworth MSc RGN SCM
Mrs E Birnie RGN
Miss Marion Buchanan RGN RSCN
Professor Christine Chapman OBE
Professor R S Downie BPhil MA
Professor A S Duncan DSC MB ChB FRCSE FRCOG FRCPE
Miss Evelyn Hide MA RGN RNT
Mr Gary Jones RGN
Dr Alison Kitson PhD RGN
Mr Harry McCree RGN RNMH
Professor Penny Prophit RN BSN MSN DNSc
Miss B M Robottom
Mrs Hazel Shaw RGN
Mrs Mary Watkins RGN RMN
Miss Sarah Whitfield RGN

1 Introduction: Ethics and Nursing

What are nurses, midwives and health visitors taught about ethics? *Teaching and Learning Nursing Ethics* is based on the findings of a study that began from this question. The study was undertaken by the Institute of Medical Ethics, in collaboration with the Royal College of Nursing, and included a major enquiry into the teaching of ethics in nursing, midwifery and health visiting* throughout the United Kingdom. The enquiry was devised by a Working Party with members from the different branches of nursing and other relevant disciplines and interests, including individuals with experience of teaching ethics. On the basis of this enquiry, the Working Party made a number of recommendations.

Further aspects of the Working Party's task were to clarify why ethical issues are now of growing professional and public interest and to examine what exactly is meant by 'ethical' issues. These questions are addressed in this chapter before turning to the study's educational findings and recommendations. The chapter begins with a brief account of some recent developments in health care, nursing and society that have contributed to greater awareness of ethical issues. It then offers some definitions of 'ethics' and related terms and discusses their relevance to the practice of nursing. This is illustrated with special reference to the principle of autonomy and the role of nursing in the health–care team.

1. BACKGROUND

Ethical issues in nursing are of growing professional and public interest. This can be seen from the increasing attention paid to them

---

* To avoid cumbersome sentences the term 'nursing' will normally be used to include midwifery and health visiting.

not only in the educational context but also in professional journals, conferences and the media. Among the more general reasons for this interest is an awareness that questions about values and moral choice are central to many developments in health care.

Against the background of a rising standard of living, biomedical and technical advances have created higher expectations of the effectiveness of health care. The prolongation of life and the relief of suffering are now commonly seen as appropriate and achievable goals. But they are not always achieved in practice and the prolongation of life is not always compatible with the relief of suffering. This can raise questions that are matters not just of clinical or political but also of moral judgment. Even when appropriate goals for health care can be agreed upon, the resources needed to achieve them are still finite. Forty years after the inception of the National Health Service (NHS), scarcity in proportion to aspiration remains an enduring feature of health care; and choices, in which the interests of some groups or individuals are inevitably at risk, continue to present themselves. Nor is it always clear, in either the political or the clinical context, who should make these choices, or how. In the clinical and administrative contexts, moreover, these problems are complicated by the fact that the boundaries of clinical responsibility are often obscured by the number of professionals and individuals involved in the care of each patient or client.

Interest in nursing ethics reflects these general developments in health care. It also reflects developments in the philosophy and practice of nursing. These have brought into focus both the distinctive role of nursing and its relations with clients and colleagues. The nurse's role as enabler and advocate, as well as health educator, has engendered an emerging professional conscience towards patients and efforts to articulate the particular logic of nursing care. In relation to other professions, especially medicine, this professional conscience has created a desire for co-operation and partnership, rather than an ancillary role in the multidisciplinary team. These developments are reflected, for example, in new codes of professional conduct (RCN, 1976; RCN, 1980; UKCC, 1984), in the introduction of the nursing process (Yura and Walsh, 1978) and in the radical review of nursing education envisaged in 'Project 2000' of the United Kingdom Central Council for Nursing, Midwifery and Health Visiting (UKCC, 1985). Not all of these developments are universally accepted within nursing or by other professions, and there is still considerable debate about the directions in which the profession should be developing. Nevertheless, the perceived growing need to articulate the logic of nursing carries with it an equal need to examine, in their own right, the ethical questions specific to nursing.

These developments in nursing and health care reflect a wider society very different from that of nursing's religious or military origins or from the time when midwifery was practised in the local community. In those earlier societies ethics was not clearly distinguished from the ethos of the group or the hierarchy. Thus, when the predecessors of modern professionals were faced with moral choices, their decisions were guided by traditional wisdom, related to the teaching of religion or the inherited precepts of their occupational group. The respected local midwife exercising her own judgment, or the nurse acting on the doctor's instructions, did so in a privacy largely protected by the mystique of her role. What happened in the patient's home, or among the poor in a religious or charity hospital, moreover, might attract some local speculation but not much wider publicity.

Today, by contrast, the moral choices of health professionals are widely discussed in the media, particularly when cases come to court or are the subject of Parliamentary questions. Consumerist claims about patients' rights, and the presence of 'whistleblowers', have made health professionals aware, in the United Kingdom and elsewhere, that their choices may be under scrutiny. Moreover, this is happening in a society much more divided than ever before in cultural, religious and moral terms. In the United Kingdom many of these divisions are obscured by the remnants of a traditional reluctance to acknowledge the influence of political or religious allegiance in many areas of public and professional life. These allegiances are customarily regarded as matters of private judgment: but their unacknowledged influence can complicate moral decision-making. Because of this, as for the other reasons suggested above, it has become important to try to analyse value judgments and moral choices in nursing and health care in the more disinterested terms of ethics.

2. 'ETHICS' AND RELATED TERMS

What exactly is meant by 'ethics'? The terms 'medical ethics', 'nursing ethics' or 'professional ethics' are familiar but can be misleading, for the word 'ethics' has various meanings and associations. First, it can refer to that branch of philosophy also called 'moral philosophy'.

Thus, philosophers write books with titles like *Methods of Ethics* or *Principia Ethica*, and such books are concerned with the study of the principles governing man's life in society. Ethics in this sense is a theoretical study of practical morality and its aim is to discover, analyse and relate to each other the fundamental concepts and principles of ordinary practical morality.

In its second main sense 'ethics' refers simply to ordinary morality, especially as it is found in a professional context. There are two reasons for preferring the terms 'moral judgment' or 'value judgment' to 'ethical judgment' in this context. The first is that using 'moral judgment' or 'value judgment' brings out the *continuity* between the moral problems encountered in hospital and those encountered in daily life and avoids the implication that there are special features about health care that require a code of behaviour different from the rest of life. The second is that the term 'ethics' encourages a narrow view of morality as consisting simply of the 'do's' and 'don'ts' of a code. It is preferable to view morality broadly as including the whole area of value judgments about 'good' and 'harm'.

In its third sense 'ethics' refers to codes, or ethics *narrowly* conceived. These codes are important, for they give some of the more general principles that underlie professional activity and they apply across cultural and national boundaries. But, clearly, basic quasi-legal principles cannot encompass the range of moral problems facing health-care professionals.

It is worthwhile stressing the difference between the second broad sense of ethics as value judgments and the narrow sense, which refers simply to items on a traditional list. For example, in a wide sense it is a moral or a value judgment that a given patient, all factors considered, ought to be allowed home despite the risk of a recurrence of his problem. But clearly this decision does not raise a question of morality or ethics narrowly conceived. When health-care professionals take ethics or morality in the narrow sense they can be unaware of the extent to which they are continually making moral or value judgments in the broad sense. There are certainly technical (both scientific and social) factors involved in deciding whether or not a given patient ought to be allowed home. But the decision about what in the end ought to be done goes beyond the technical and encompasses the professional's overall judgment as to what is for the total good of the patient. This overall, all-things-considered judgment of the patient's good is what is meant by a moral or a value judgment.

In order to understand the ethics of nursing then, particular attention needs to be paid to the all-pervasive nature of moral and value judgments. Value judgments are judgments about what is most important to us (what we prize, value or cherish) and hence what we choose above other things; our values, ultimately, are what motivate and move us. But a problem about values is that, in many situations, we rarely value only one thing. In the case mentioned in the previous paragraph, for example, both the patient's general health (which might best be served by keeping him in hospital) and his autonomy or self-determination (which might be served, if that is what he wishes, by allowing him home) may be valued. There may then be a conflict of values, which, in extreme cases, can become a moral dilemma – a problem that cannot be resolved without offending against one of the values involved. True moral dilemmas are not very common since long before they can arise an accumulation of everyday value judgments have often predetermined the issue. But precisely because of this, examining moral dilemmas has the important educational function of clarifying what is at stake in everyday moral or value judgments.

Conflicts may arise simply between different values prized by one individual, or between personal and professional values, or again between any of these and the values of a particular patient or of society. A variety of psychologically-orientated techniques has been devised in order to help individuals gain greater understanding of what their own values actually are (Goldman and Arbuthnot, 1979). But if these techniques are then used to advocate a particular hierarchy of values (arguing that certain values are more important than others), this further step may be questionable, since any such hierarchy itself represents a value judgment. It may be, of course, the responsibility of professional bodies or educational institutions to maintain a hierarchy of value-based standards or principles. But it is important to realise that these are arrived at, not by some objective scientific process, but through intersubjective agreement, often of a political nature. Thus, while there is a proper place in professional education for teaching the ethical standards of the profession, this does not preclude critical ethical examination of the reasons for and against these standards and the values on which they are based.

3. ETHICAL PRINCIPLES

This brief introduction will not list or analyse in any detail the variety of ethical issues that arise in everyday nursing practice. As has already been suggested, these issues relate to moral choices about the best interests of patients and others, to conflicts of duty, loyalty and the nurse's professional and personal conscience, to value choices made in management, research and policy decisions, and to value preferences engendered in nursing education. These issues in turn raise more general ethical questions, including those of rights, paternalism, autonomy, advocacy and accountability. The interface between ethical issues and questions of communication is also relevant in this context, since the two are commonly interrelated, as were ethics and etiquette in the past.

To illustrate the relevance of ethics to everyday nursing practice it may suffice at this point simply to make some comments about the implications, for practice and teamwork, of the ethical principle of *respect for autonomy*. Respect for autonomy is one of the three major principles that, according to many commentators, sum up the ideals of health-care ethics expressed in most professional codes and declarations on the subject. The two remaining principles are those of *justice, or fairness, and beneficence and non-maleficence*.

The principle of beneficence and non-maleficence (in other words the duty to do good and not harm) was the cornerstone of traditional medical ethics, particularly as long as the doctor's therapeutic effectiveness largely depended on the confidence he was able to inspire in his special knowledge and skill. In this context, the unequal nature of the doctor–patient relationship focused attention on the doctor's responsibilities for his patient's interests. More recently, however, thinking in both philosophy and health care has balanced against this the need to emphasise the patient's wishes. This emphasis has been a feature of modern moral philosophy since its origins in the eighteenth century. In health care it has grown with the realisation of medicine's increasing technical ability to do both good and harm.

This increasing ability to do harm as well as good often demands, in response, value judgments as well as clinical judgments. Because of this, the need to consult the patient's wishes has come to be seen as increasingly important. Respect for autonomy (the individual's right, or liberty, to choose) has thus emerged as a principle of both moral and therapeutic significance. But this has created other centres of decision-making alongside those involving medical beneficence, and this in turn raises the possibility of conflicting choices related to the interests and wishes of different patients, nurses, doctors and others. In this context the principle of justice or fairness obviously has also to be emphasised in order to mediate among conflicting claims.

Emphasis on respect for autonomy has also led to emphasis on informed consent to treatment and on the obligations of patients to co-operate with those caring for them. In health care, of course, most patients are normally dependent to some degree on health workers and, with this in mind, the idea of a 'fiduciary relationship' of trust and negotiation has been suggested as an alternative to traditional paternalism. But since, as a matter of justice, the autonomy of carers as well as of those in their care has to be respected, such relationships should reflect realism about the powers as well as the limitations of professionals.

4. PRINCIPLES AND PRACTICE

Giving due weight to each of the three major principles of health care in this way has practical implications for the roles of the different professions, particularly within health teams working in partnership with patients. This can be illustrated with reference to some different areas of health care.

4.1 Chronic illness and old age

In relation to chronic illness, old age and self-inflicted disorders, the proper role of the nurse is clearly as a complementary partner to the doctor and patient. There is no longer any justification for the role of handmaid to the doctor. The need, rather, is for a competent practitioner with specified areas of expertise and responsibility.

Against this background areas of nursing care that are tried and tested, reliable and effective, and preferably research-based can rightly be 'claimed' by nurses for the benefit of patients. Among these areas are, for example; psychological care to prevent and alleviate the distress of patients and relatives; helping patients and relatives with practical problems related to illness; and providing symptom relief and comfort. Confirmation by patients and other staff that nurses are expected to have the expertise to fulfil these functions should encourage such care to be given.

In this context, too, there is a great need for nurses to become preventative agents, helping people to give up unhealthy forms of behaviour, identifying health risks, and reducing the secondary morbidity consequent on certain chronic conditions. Moreover, the larger proportion of very frail elderly in society justifies the provision of more care to alleviate and prevent problems related to morale, weakness and diminished abilities. For nurses in these areas to achieve some independence of practice, their knowledge and skill must be established, standards must be clearly identified and achievable, and others must recognise their areas of independence. Above all, individual nurses must be willing to accept responsibility for providing necessary care and feel accountable for success and failure.

4.2 Acute illness

There are other areas of nursing and medicine, where roles are intrinsically linked: teamwork involves interdependence and shared knowledge as well as distinct contributions. Various factors affect this degree of interdependence, many relating to the patient's situation, others pertaining to a lack of understanding and respect among staff.

Acute areas with emergency and highly invasive interventions tend to militate against independent roles for the doctor and nurse who work in such close confines, intensively dealing with similar problems of life-threatening proportions, such as blood pressure control, blood gas maintenance, fluid balance and ventilation. This type of partnership depends on an individual's competence and on personal aspects of trust, mutual referral and delegation. Anyone who has witnessed intensive care staff will realise that roles do tend to overlap to a great extent and that patients need so much help that they often lose all thought of independent action or choice, at least in the most acute phases.

4.3 The general hospital

In other areas, such as the general hospital, the picture is rather different. Frequently, nursing roles are poorly defined and competencies are ignored. Areas of nursing expertise need to be promoted and integrated into practice but organisational constraints reduce opportunities. Nurses complain that they have to run the service and have inadequate time to care for patients. Patients are introduced into the busy hospital bureaucracy and suffer much anxiety and frustration through lack of information and opportunity to make decisions. This picture could be avoided if staff, particularly nurses, formed a truly professional relationship with patients. Problem-orientated care, based on full and open communication and a systematic assessment of need, reflecting the patient's preferences, as negotiated with them, producing shared goals for care, would be ideal in terms of the principles discussed earlier. There is some evidence that this is developing in the United Kingdom, even if, in the past, patients and their families were too conditioned into accepting a passive role.

4.4 Primary care

Primary care, by contrast, offers greater autonomy for patients and greater professional independence for nurses. Although community care is far from ideal in many areas, especially the inner cities, individuals' needs and the context of care are less dependent on institutional bureaucracy. The introduction of innovative roles, such as that of the nurse practitioner, in some places has demonstrated the usefulness of greater independence for the nurse in terms of the contribution she can make to health care. Individuals have been shown to seek access to the nurse practitioner predominantly for health education, child rearing, advice on caring for an elderly relative, counselling for 'worries' and advice on managing practical problems related to chronic illness. General practitioners are realising that their own expertise can be employed more efficiently in areas of medical diagnosis and treatment and that they can refer many patients and families with more general health-related problems to the nurse practitioner.

4.5 Independence, accountability and autonomy

Such independence, however, can flourish only if the nurse is prepared to be totally accountable and culpable for her own care. Legally, she would require professional status, clearly defined areas of practice, and, of course, indemnity insurance. (Problems with this kind of arrangement, it might be noted, are currently arising in North America, where insurance premiums are equivalent to a major proportion of the salary. These might not arise so acutely in the United Kingdom but would require to be monitored so that adequate ways of resolving them in the general interest of both nurses and patients might be found.)

Within the 'progressive' team-work setting sketched above, relationships between professional carers and with clients shift quite clearly towards the partnership model, with each participant having personal autonomy and a sphere of independence. Today there is evidence that traditional relationships within the health-care team (in which the doctor automatically determined not only the content of the work, but also the manner in which it was done) are, in fact, disappearing. This change is occurring because other team members are beginning to assert their rights and because the pace and quantity of work is increasing in most practices and specialties.

4.6 Organisational factors

In the face of increasing demand, a shortage of nurses is a particularly critical factor. It means that they must only be used for those functions which require their expertise. Nurses are thus in a position to be much more assertive in deciding where they should direct their greatest and most effective energies. Others who have less specific preparation are taking on clerical and administrative tasks. Their presence, however, affects the working of any team, making it more complex, and necessitating even more care with communication.

In the institutional setting, although all members of staff are employed by the health authority, different members may be answerable to different 'bosses'. Nurses still work in a linear relationship from the ward level to macro-organisational levels of nursing. In reality, nurse managers have little control over patient care, tending to manage nurses rather than patients, while maintaining responsibility for providing resources for clinical care. Nevertheless, nurse managers have often been used by nurses as a barrier to legitimate the development of more independence. Conflict between the hierarchical pattern of a managed service and a professional, autonomous pattern is becoming less problematic as nurse managers now tend to be used for advice rather than 'control', and as the professional service that nurses provide is seen to justify proper rewards, recognition and resources.

4.7 The relationship between nurse, doctor and patient

The nurse–doctor relationship is also changing as nurses progress from the image of doctor's handmaiden to independent practitioner. In certain settings, for example the nurse-run services provided by the Oxford Health Authority, this has proved highly successful. Doctors and nurses make referrals to one another, and the patients for whom primary responsibility rests with the nurse tend to be those who need rehabilitation or are elderly and need some help with coping at home.

In this setting, patients are assigned to one primary nurse, an arrangement similar to that in medicine. The nurse assesses needs with the patient and his relatives (or significant others), plans and evaluates care and is accountable for the outcome. In this way a complementary partnership between doctor and nurse really is possible, with neither being answerable or superior to the other. Many of these features are similar to those found in some terminal care settings, where maximising choice and respecting autonomy are encouraged. In each of these settings, however, nurses may tend to offer unlimited commitment in order to provide 24-hour cover and some need to recognise their own rights as well as those of their patients.

In the patient-team relationship there are many dimensions, from the therapeutic duo to the need for multiple services provided by many people for the patient and his family members. Incumbent on the patient are those obligations involved in the fiduciary principle, such as providing information and the willingness to negotiate and agree on certain choices and goals. Realistic contracts based on reciprocity are also essential in promoting healthy forms of behaviour. This type of agreement involves true participation, based on a clear exposition of facts and preferences. In this context doctors and nurses become less prescriptive and may have to reduce their expectations of perfect results or ideal treatment plans in return for promises made by the patient. Consultations tend to resemble counselling sessions, in which patients are helped to work through problems in order to ameliorate them, specific medical information being offered as necessary. This degree of involvement is also frequently encouraged in the self-help group setting, sometimes arranged by staff but rarely 'led' by them.

When dealing with the team more complex working arrangements may be involved for the patient and his family. The client may in fact help to co-ordinate his own health care by keeping drug or co-operation cards. It is vital that all members of the team share treatment goals and that less helpful tendencies (for example, when one member contradicts another or is manipulated within a complex relationship) be avoided. In this setting the patient has the right to all relevant services if he agrees to plans for care and helps with communication and co-ordination.

5. PRACTICE, ETHICS AND LOGIC

The developments discussed above are simply one way of illustrating the relevance of an ethical principle such as that of autonomy to the practical aspects of everyday nursing. Other related ethical issues, such as those of confidentiality, truth-telling and resource allocation, are of no less practical significance. These, and many others, are issues with which ethics is concerned and which it can help clarify. Nursing practice also raises questions with which the study (traditionally associated with ethics) of logic is concerned. The introduction of the nursing process and care plans as an attempt to achieve more individualised care for patients, for example, requires logical thinking as well as an ability to justify moral choices. As patients and their families become involved in relationships of greater partnership with health professionals, education in moral reasoning and logical thinking alike will become a prime requirement for nursing.

2 | Why Teach Ethics?

Many ethical issues are raised by the practice of nursing. How should nursing education respond to this? The reply of most nurse educators is that the study of ethics should be part of the curriculum. In response to the Institute of Medical Ethics (IME) questionnaire (see Appendix I) over 98% (n = 147) of those responsible for basic nursing education said this, as did a similar proportion of those teaching midwives, health visitors and district nurses. All respondents responsible for intensive therapy courses stated that ethics should be part of these courses, and the need to deal with ethical issues in post-basic and continuing education was emphasised by almost all the tutors responding from that area.

Such near-unanimity of response may suggest to the sceptical that being in favour of ethics teaching is like being in favour of virtue – a sentiment so vague that everyone can agree with it. Being in favour of virtue, in fact, does seem to provide one of the more general motives for advocating ethics teaching. But more particular reasons can be, and were, stated by the respondents to the IME questionnaire. This chapter examines these reasons and asks what objectives they imply for ethics teaching.

Responses to the IME questionnaire suggest that those responsible for nursing education envisage at least four different reasons for teaching ethics. The most commonly expressed reason was that nurses need to understand ethics in order to practise professionally. The second reason was that nurses need to understand their own and other people's 'value systems'. The third was that nurses 'need to learn to reason', and the fourth that 'nursing is humanitarian in nature'.

On examination these reasons for teaching ethics seem, at different points, both to overlap and to be in conflict with each other. The most obvious areas of overlap are between the first and third reasons (professionalism and reasoning) and between the second and fourth (values and humanitarianism), while the most obvious tension is between these pairs. The tension might be characterised as having to do with a difference between thinking and feeling, and the implications of this for educational objectives may thus be quite complicated. But before attempting an overview of the implied aims and objectives the two pairs of reasons should be examined in greater detail, drawing out the implications of each.

1. PROFESSIONALISM

As already stated, the most commonly expressed reason for ethics teaching was to enable nurses to practise professionally. As one (basic/general; B/G) respondent put it, 'all nursing decisions have an ethical component', but 'many nurses are not aware of the ethical implications of what they are doing'. This lack of awareness of such 'a key priority for the caring professions', another (B/G) argues, had its historical roots in nursing's 'institutionalised parochialism', which avoided 'the challenge of ethical discussion and debate'. This, clearly, was not appropriate to the independent professional stance of contemporary nursing. 'We should encourage nurses', a third (B/G) respondent wrote, 'to question the ethical nature of some of the practices taking place in medicine and nursing today'. It was necessary, the respondent went on, 'to help nurses to exercise professional judgment'. A further (post-basic; P/B) respondent agreed:

> If a qualified nurse is to continue to develop professionally, she needs to be able to understand how ethical decision–making works, so that she can have confidence to join in the debate . . . .

Seen in this way, as a matter of professionalism, the reason for ethics teaching is not dissimilar to the reason for codes of ethics or professional conduct. In either case the profession's specific responsibilities and their limits are being defined and clarified. This was reflected in one (midwifery; M) respondent's general remark that 'there must be a perimeter within which to work'. Other respondents mentioned nursing responsibilities and their limits with particular reference to the law, to patients and clients and to other professionals. In relation to the first of these, one (P/B) noted that 'professional discipline and litigation' now form 'part of our working lives', while another (M) argued that ethics should be taught as a result 'of the move towards defensive practice because of litigation problems'.
Defensiveness was certainly not a characteristic of many responses

concerning professionalism towards patients or clients. Another respondent (M) even went so far as to say that 'the main reason' for including ethics teaching in the curriculum was 'to allow women and partners to have a real say in what happens to them during pregnancy, delivery and afterwards'. A similar emphasis on the rights and personal freedom of patients (together with some reference to advocacy) was expressed by respondents from intensive therapy, and mental handicap and mental nursing, the latter with special reference to compulsory treatment.

With reference to nursing's relations with other professions, the protection of patients, as well as of staff, was also cited as a reason for ethics teaching. One respondent (M) saw a need 'to curb medical or surgical enthusiasts and keep the interests of patients paramount'. This remark was made with special reference to research: the respondent was concerned about 'preventing the ends justifying the means and research for research's sake'.

2. REASONING

Respondents were concerned to encourage a professional approach to nursing and, in its relation to formal responsibility, to patients, clients and other professions. Ethics teaching was seen as a prerequisite for this in at least three ways. One was simply in terms of awareness of the existence of ethical issues. The criticism (B/G) that 'many nurses are not aware of the ethical implications of what they are doing' has already been noted. It was complemented by a respondent (P/B) who wrote:

> Ethics, like politics, is part of life. It is important for all nurses, particularly those on post-basic courses, to be aware and knowledgeable in this area.

This need for awareness was echoed by a further (continuing education; C/E) respondent:

> All students should be aware of the ethical dilemmas of life while working in the community and responsible for decisions.

A similar response (M) stated that ethics teaching was important because 'a person should be informed widely so that he can make an analytical and valued judgment'.

As this last statement suggests, ethics teaching was seen to be of

value not only in creating awareness of the issues but also in helping
nurses, as an intensive therapy (IT) respondent put it, 'to cope
effectively with some of the ethical and moral dilemmas they encounter'. Ethics teaching was thus necessary in the view of a (B/G)
respondent:

> because nurses need to learn to reason, to put forward an argument
> and make moral decisions when confronted by conflict in their daily
> practice.

In addition to creating awareness of ethical issues, and teaching how
to reason about them, ethics teaching was seen as providing a moral
basis for nursing practice. One respondent (M) put it like this:

> the complex and pluralist society within which we function de-
> mands the ability to be consistent in decision-making. A sound
> knowledge of principles of ethics should assist in this.

A not dissimilar response (IT) elaborated this point by suggesting that
'advocacy could be viewed as the philosophical foundation of nursing,
based on common humanity, needs and human rights'.

3. AIMS AND OBJECTIVES IMPLIED

What educational aims and objectives are implied in this first pair of
reasons for teaching ethics to nurses? The following might be
suggested:

1. To create an awareness of ethical issues in nursing.
2. To develop an understanding of:

    a. the principles of ethics;
    b. the philosophical foundations of nursing;
    c. the legal and disciplinary responsibilities and constraints of
        nursing practice.

3. To help students learn:

    a. to reason;
    b. to analyse the ethical issues;
    c. to put forward arguments;
    d. to understand ethical decision-making.

4. To give nurses confidence in:

    a. exercising professional judgment;

    b. questioning the ethics of medical or nursing practices;

    c. making moral decisions;

    d. being advocates of patient autonomy.

5. To enable nurses to cope more effectively with some of the ethical and moral dilemmas they encounter.

4. ILLUSTRATION: RESEARCH

The aims and objectives implied by the first pair of reasons for teaching ethics clearly create a formidable agenda for ethics teaching. Furthermore, aims and objectives may be inferred from the second pair of reasons. But before considering these it may be useful to illustrate the aims and objectives so far with an example mentioned by one respondent, namely the ethics of research. How may this be dealt with in ethics teaching?

The initial aim, 'to create awareness of ethical issues in nursing', may be met by discussing case studies of the moral dilemmas that can arise when nurses are involved in the process of obtaining consent for medical or nursing research or when nursing students are undertaking educational projects. The very least that might be expected of this would be, for example, to dispel any notion that patients consent merely by virtue of their status as patients.

In order to meet the second set of aims and objectives (i.e. to develop an understanding of the principles of ethics, etc.) it would be necessary to discuss:

1. the relevance to research of general ethical principles such as:

   - informed consent, autonomy and respect for persons;
   - beneficence and non-maleficence;
   - utility, and evaluating harms and benefits;
   - justice or fairness in selecting subjects;

2. the philosophical implications of nursing as a caring but also knowledge-based profession;

3. relevant legal and disciplinary considerations, mentioning, for example, what the law requires in terms of consent from patients who are competent or incompetent.

The third set of aims and objectives (concerned with reasoning, analysing, putting forward arguments and understanding ethical decision-making) again might be met through case-study analysis.

Included here may be situations in which, for example, the patient's comprehension of what is involved in the research is in doubt or the nurse has doubts about the potential benefits of the study or the possible risks of the procedures involved, or again, if the nurse experiences conflict between the care-giving and consent-seeking roles. In discussing such cases, students may be asked to state an opinion about what ought to be done, give reasons for this and consider counter-arguments, or whether their reasons would still hold good if the crucial features of the case or the context were different. Such features as the degree of invasiveness of the procedures involved, the age of the patient, or the seriousness of the condition or the problem being investigated, for example, may be changed.

Discussion intended to meet the third set of aims and objectives should seek to identify the moral features of the case and, through argument, counter-argument and consideration of other cases, make explicit the moral distinctions and concepts which different cases share. Examining and clarifying these distinctions and concepts, and seeing how they relate to one another, can lead, in turn, to a discussion of the more abstract issues mentioned above in relation to the second set of aims and objectives. Introduction of these more abstract issues at this later, rather than earlier, point may thus make them seem more relevant and of greater interest to the students.

Whether these more abstract issues are introduced at an earlier or later point is likely to depend on a number of contingent factors. If the aim is to ensure that the maximum number of relevant moral principles, philosophical concepts and legal or disciplinary requirements is presented to the students in the time available, a series of lectures on moral philosophy and law would seem to be required. On the other hand, unless these subjects are components of an academic degree course, there may be insufficient time available for lectures in the relevant theoretical issues to do more than impart 'a little knowledge', which is proverbially dangerous. The alternative is to introduce some account of these issues as they arise, for example, to say 'What we have been doing so far is almost exclusively using what philosophers call Utilitarian and Consequentialist arguments. These are not the only kinds of argument that can be used about this kind of case.' Some discussion of the different types of moral argument can then be introduced. This approach may of course sacrifice comprehensiveness to relevance, but in the time available it may be the preferable option. To use this 'Socratic' approach successfully, however, the teacher needs to have a confident and informed grasp of the philosophical issues and also a good rapport with the students.

The fourth and fifth sets of aims and objectives stated above, of course, go well beyond the ability of ethics teaching to influence directly. Ethics teaching, however, has traditionally been seen as part of the basic education of the learned (or knowledge-based) professions, particularly as a mental discipline preparing students for mature, balanced and confident decision-making. In the twentieth century, of course, ethics teaching has played a much less prominent role in the education of the scientific professions, including medicine. But, equally, as ethical problems in science and medicine become more prominent, so the lack of ethics teaching is increasingly being regretted and remedied. The near-unanimous view that ethics should be part of the nursing curriculum would thus seem to belong to the contemporary development of nursing as an independent and knowledge-based profession.

5. VALUES AND HUMANITARIANISM

Nurses are not only professionals but also people – individuals, each with experience and views of their own. The second pair of reasons for the teaching of ethics, mentioned by the respondents to the IME questionnaire, reflects this. As one (B/G) argues:

> It is essential that nurse learners have an opportunity to explore ethical problems related to their own system of values and to the values of others – patients or clients and peers.

Another respondent (C/E) expressed a similar view:

> The basis of decision-making in nursing, midwifery and health visiting is rooted in the value systems and beliefs of the practitioners.

Respondents from most areas of nursing, midwifery and health visiting echoed these views.

Alongside this emphasis on understanding values was the fourth reason for teaching ethics. This was commonly referred to in relation to what one (P/B) respondent described as 'humanitarian factors', and the point was made by another (B/G), who wrote that:

> Nursing is humanitarian in nature, which involves ethical and moral dilemmas.

Advocating ethics teaching with reference to values and humanitarianism suggests a shorter but no less significant set of educational aims and objectives. The next chapter will examine how far these and the objectives summarised earlier match the objectives actually stated by respondents and the topics covered by the courses. But at this point, again, what are the educational objectives implied by the second pair of reasons given for ethics teaching?

6. HUMANITARIAN OBJECTIVES

The argument that nursing 'involves ethical and moral dilemmas' because 'it is humanitarian in nature' is perhaps the most general reason for teaching ethics and also the most difficult from which to infer particular objectives. Dictionary definitions of 'humanitarian' are a distinct disadvantage here, since they suggest that the word implies having a regard (perhaps excessive or hypocritical) for the interests of the entire human race. The general sense of the argument, however, is perhaps clear enough to sum it up by returning to terminology used earlier: that is, the aim implied might be to encourage nurses to act according to the principles of respect for persons, beneficence and non-maleficence, and justice.

This aim, however, does not entirely sum up what seems to be implied by the word 'humanitarian', since it suggests not only acting according to these principles but also being *disposed* to act according to them. This additional factor goes well beyond the aims and objectives inferred from the earlier pair of reasons (which were concerned in the main with clear thinking) and into the realm of feeling. In other words, it moves the discussion from the traditional concerns of ethics or moral philosophy to those of *moral education*. An obvious difficulty about this, however, mentioned in the previous chapter, is the disputable value of any attempt to spell out the aims of moral education: for example, which of the principles mentioned above should take precedence when there is conflict between them? This difficulty is complicated, moreover, by cultural and religious differences. An example of the latter is the view of some Jewish thinkers that the value of human life makes divulging a fatal diagnosis to a patient something that requires justification. Many other moral thinkers, by contrast, would hold that respect for autonomy makes not divulging such a diagnosis require justification.

The aims and objectives implied by the 'humanitarian values' of nursing would thus appear to be counsel for perfection, which belongs to the sphere of personal morality rather than nursing ethics. This conclusion, however, cannot be entirely the end of the matter since in practice there are two ways in which this widely held reason for teaching ethics can be expressed in terms of acceptable educational aims and objectives. One of these can be brought out more clearly by discussing the argument that nurses need to understand their own and other people's 'value systems'. This is discussed in the next section. The other relates to the codes of conduct and disciplinary procedures of the nursing profession.

The existence of codes of conduct and disciplinary procedures in nursing, it may be argued, is an expression of the fact that nursing is 'humanitarian in nature', that is, if nursing did not share the 'humanitarian' ideals of the other caring professions, many ethical issues might not arise from it. Even in the public relations of commerce and business, after all, some agreed ethics of truth–telling and trustworthiness is necessary. But this is particularly important for a profession such as nursing, which requires its members, in the words of the UKCC Code of Professional Conduct (UKCC, 1984), to:

> act in such a manner as to justify public trust and confidence, to uphold and enhance the good standing and reputation of the profession, to serve the public interest and the interests of the patients/clients.

Beginning from the humanitarian nature of nursing as a reason for teaching ethics, then, an implied educational aim would be:

> to commend to students the profession's own standards of conduct, competence and caring.

This objective differs from item 2c (p. 16) ('to develop an understanding of the legal and disciplinary responsibilities and constraints of nursing practice') since it is concerned not only with describing but also with *commending* these standards. It is concerned, moreover, with commending not only minimum standards but also those of professional excellence.

This, clearly, is not an aim that can be confined to ethics teaching if the latter is seen as a subject separable from the rest of nursing education. It is, rather, an aspect of all nursing education and an aim for all teachers. Commending professional excellence in standards of conduct, competence and caring is a task to be achieved not by making rhetorical statements but by attending to the small details of attitudes, practices and interactions. This aim, therefore, is particularly important for teachers in the clinical area who, like those using the 'Socratic' approach mentioned earlier, will succeed only in proportion to the confidence with which they grasp the details of the standards concerned and the quality of their rapport with their students.

It may, of course, be objected here that commending professional excellence is not really a matter of ethics but of practice. This objection may be raised when ethics is regarded primarily as a matter of moral dilemmas or major choices. Against this view, the philosopher Iris Murdoch (Murdoch, 1985) has argued cogently:

> If we consider what the work of attention is like, how continuously it goes on, and how imperceptively it builds up structures of value around us, we shall not be surprised that at crucial moments of choice most of the business of choosing is already over. This does not imply that we are not free, certainly not.
>
> But it implies that the exercise of our freedom is a small piecemeal business which goes on all the time and not a grandiose leaping about unimpeded at important moments. The moral life, in this view, is something that goes on continually.

'To commend the profession's own standards of conduct, competence and caring' is thus an aim of all nursing education and not simply of ethics teaching as a subject separable from the remainder. When curricular time is specifically identified for ethics teaching, however, one way of meeting the aim would be to examine a current code of conduct (such as that of the UKCC) in relation to examples of the matters with which it is concerned. This will provide an opportunity to identify different ways in which the statements of the codes might be interpreted, including exceptional cases and conflicting interpretations. The concepts employed in the statements may also be traced back to the ethical principles from which they derive.

Such an examination of a code, of course, might equally well be undertaken to meet item 2c, p. 16, and in that context (of 'clear thinking') the standards of the profession would be regarded as, in principle, themselves open to question on ethical grounds. In specifically identified ethics teaching there will be a greater opportunity to go into such questions than in, say, teaching in the clinical area. Such questioning, it may be superfluous to add, need not be regarded as going against the aim of commending the profession's standards since, precisely by questioning them, the reasons why the profession has espoused them may become clearer.

7. VALUE SYSTEMS

What aims and objectives are implied by the argument that ethics should be taught because nurses need to understand their own and others' 'value systems'? Two different sets of aims and objectives would seem to be implied here: the first concerned with thinking and reasoning, the second with feelings, emotions and attitudes. A distinction of this kind is suggested by the fact that respondents to the IME questionnaire chose to speak about 'value systems' rather than simply 'values'.

The term 'value systems' implies some degree of explicit organisation in how people think about what they value. The degree to which individuals consciously organise their values, however, varies considerably and changes with time and experience. Thus, there is no simple method whereby nurses can learn to understand the value systems of other individuals. However, it is possible for nurses to become informed about values that appear to be significant to different sections of society or groups within it. Such information can be provided either by the social sciences or from what the most organised groups themselves profess as their values.

This information is of obvious importance today since nurses and patients alike now come from a great variety of different backgrounds. Relevant differences here include not only those of ethnic origin or religious belief but also those arising from the fact that the increasing proportion of elderly patients or clients has beliefs, attitudes and values formed in a very different world from that familiar to nursing students today. In the United Kingdom regional, rural/urban and social class differences also may be responsible for different values, and the capacity of members of the different sexes to misunderstand what really matters to those of the other is, of course, universal.

How much responsibility should ethics teaching assume for providing information relevant to these differences? Providing information about all of these differences is clearly a task beyond the capacity of teachers of nursing or nursing ethics, who by definition are not teachers of comparative religion and culture. On the other hand, mature teachers of nursing will be aware of significant differences in cultural, religious, political or generation values related to such matters as the human body, privacy, family relationships, pain, termination of pregnancy and ways of addressing other people. If the professed or observed values of different social groups about such matters are not discussed elsewhere in nursing education, clearly ethics teaching has a responsibility to provide some information about them. The objective here, therefore, would be:

> to provide information about significant differences in the professed or observed values of different ethnic, cultural, religious, political, generational and other groups.

Providing information, however, does not entirely exhaust the meaning of 'understanding' the values of other people. What values mean to the individual or group who hold them is not necessarily the same as what they mean to the outside observer. The latter, inevitably, understands other people's values in terms of his own, and this is the case even when the observer is trying as much as possible to be 'value-free' or 'non-judgmental', since these attitudes themselves reflect values. To advocate 'understanding' of other people's values (particularly in the context of teaching ethics to members of a humanitarian profession) thus implies commending imaginative and empathic understanding and this, it can be argued, is most likely to be found in individuals who have a mature understanding of their own values. These individuals are less likely to feel threatened by values with which they may disagree and hence are more likely to be able to use their imagination about how others feel.

These considerations suggest the following aim:

> to commend to students:
> a. a mature understanding of their own values;
> b. imaginative and empathic understanding of the values of others.

The aim here, it may be noted, is that such understanding should be commended to students, not that it should be possessed by them. The obvious reasons for this are not only the practical problems of assessing this kind of understanding but also that, in principle, any such assessment would have to be based on contestable value judgments. The advice 'know thyself' (displayed in the Temple at Delphi) is one of the first pieces of philosophical wisdom. But philosophers, not to mention psychologists, theologians and anyone who thinks about this matter, define self-understanding in too many different ways for any single definition of it to be generally accepted. Perhaps the only thing that most thinkers might agree upon is that although self-understanding is extremely difficult to achieve, the attempt to achieve it is of supreme importance. Much the same, it seems likely, would be agreed about the importance of trying to understand other people.

This aim, then, it may seem, is likely to command agreement in proportion to its lack of definition of what constitutes understanding of self, others and their respective values. The conclusion might thus be drawn that the aim is simply rhetorical and of little practical guidance. Against this, however, it may be argued that much of the work of defining what constitutes 'understanding' must be done by the students themselves. This is because, as has already been suggested, no-one else can understand an individual (although they may understand aspects of that individual) better than the individual him or herself. Commending understanding is thus a matter of encouraging and challenging students to do this work of understanding their own understanding and of each being his or her own final arbiter of its success, which will be measured not just in the classroom but in his or her own professional and other spheres of life.

The interpretation of this aim has at least three practical implications. The first is that teachers should be seen to respect the moral views of students even when the teachers do not agree with these. Such respect is best expressed in the working assumption that students normally have reasons for their moral views, and that if these reasons can be made explicit, good arguments both for and against these views can normally be found. It is important, in other words, for the teacher to get across from the outset that there are no unquestionably 'right' or 'wrong' answers to ethical questions.

A second practical implication relates to some moral questions, of which abortion is an obvious example, on which conflicting views are strongly held and the argument advanced that these are too 'personal' to be discussed in the classroom. If students (or, as is sometimes the case, teachers) are unwilling to discuss such subjects, their reticence must be respected. But before the attempt to discuss them is abandoned, the point should be made that precisely because opinion is so strongly divided there are probably good arguments for the view held by the person who is unwilling to discuss it, and that his or her view might actually be strengthened by having to become better acquainted with these arguments.

Sometimes, of course, the arguments that these views are too 'personal' to discuss may mean that the student's views are based on religious beliefs or some other world view that he or she does not want to discuss in this context. Here again, reticence must be respected, but again the point may be made that most religious and other organised world views advance philosophical as well as theological or ideological reasons for their moral opinions and, moreover, do this in the arena of public discussion. In this context, especially, it is important for teachers to show that one can respect moral opinions without necessarily agreeing with them.

The third practical implication may also be related to the discussion of such sensitive topics. A further reason for discussing these subjects in the educational context, it might be suggested, is that conflicting views on them are held not only by nurses but also by patients. An ability to articulate and criticise the relevant moral arguments on different sides of these questions may thus create a better awareness of the strengths of arguments with which one does not agree, and this in turn may lead to greater respect for those who hold them.

In this context, it may be observed, the values implicit in the behaviour and attitudes of different nurses and patients are sometimes so different that what seems important to one is not even apparent to another. In ethics teaching, therefore, it may be helpful to explore in some detail aspects of what students are tempted to label as 'irrational' behaviour or unreasonable emotions in patients or colleagues. This may help students to become aware not only of the values of others but also of their own, together with the attendant emotions that prove that these are values and not simply opinions.

8. SUMMARY

This chapter has looked at the reasons for teaching ethics to nurses given by the respondents to the IME questionnaire, and it has asked what aims and objectives for ethics teaching are implied by these reasons. Of the eight identified, some are really general aims or even aspirations, while the remainder are of different kinds. Some, for example, are concerned with thinking and reasoning, others with feelings, emotions and attitudes; again, some are concerned with professional values and others with personal. One of the main differences, however, is between those which are the concern of all nursing education and those which seem to require some special activity labelled 'ethics teaching'. In some cases this distinction is not clear and there are areas of overlap, but in order to see what is being expected of ethics teaching, it may be helpful to look again at the aims and objectives identified in the light of this distinction.

The most general aim among those identified is:

to enable nurses to cope more effectively with some of the ethical and moral dilemmas they encounter.

This aim provides a reason for teaching ethics in the context of nursing education but says little about the nature or content of such teaching.

More specific is:

> to give nurses confidence in:
> a. exercising professional judgment;
> b. questioning the ethics of medical and nursing practices;
> c. making moral decisions;
> d. being advocates of patient autonomy.

Here again, however, little is said about how this aim is to be achieved. Both of these aims, then, are perhaps best seen as belonging to nursing education in general, as is:

> to commend to students the profession's own standards of context, competence and caring.

If these aims are those of the nurse's professional education generally, by the same token they are those of ethics teaching in that context. Insofar as they specify matters of ethics, moreover, they suggest that these should be dealt with explicitly in nursing education. More specific advice on how ethics should be taught is given in the following aim and sets of objectives:

> to commend to students:
> a. a mature understanding of their own values;
> b. imagination and empathic understanding of the values of others;

> to develop an understanding of:
> a. the principles of ethics;
> b. the philosophical foundations of nursing;
> c. the legal and disciplinary responsibilities and constraints of nursing practice;

> to help students learn:
> a. to reason;
> b. to analyse ethical issues;
> c. to put forward arguments;
> d. to understand ethical decision-making.

The two sets of objectives ('to develop an understanding of' and 'help students learn') are concerned in the main with thinking and reasoning. What they suggest is required is something not very different from the nature and content of moral philosophy, applied to nursing practice, together with some knowledge of relevant aspects of law and professional discipline. In the same teaching context, if not dealt with elsewhere, a further intellectual component is required 'to provide information about significant differences in the professed or observed values of different ethnic, cultural, religious, political, generational and other groups'.

If these objectives, together with the more general preliminary aim (to create an awareness of critical issues in nursing), summed up all that was expected from ethics teaching, the needs could be met by applying the methods of moral philosophy in the context of nursing education. Something of this kind, along the lines sketched earlier in this chapter, clearly seems to be needed and possible, given curricular time and appropriately trained teachers. But in the context of nursing education, no less clearly, an additional aim seems to be called for, one concerned with feelings, emotions and attitudes and focused on values. As has been suggested earlier in this chapter, it is very difficult indeed to make specific recommendations about how this aim should be implemented in practice, and although a number of practical suggestions have been made, they are no more than suggestions. It may be, here as elsewhere in life, that the most important questions are those on which it is most difficult to reach precise agreement. It also seems to be in the nature of professionalism itself that ethical questions demand not just an intellectual but an individual emotional response. This is because, as a member of another profession has written, 'the word "professional" means that "I am responsible to myself" '. But how far this additional component is something that respondents to the IME questionnaire were able to identify and suggest ways of implementing will be identified in the next chapter.

3 Course Objectives and Content

1. OBJECTIVES

The previous chapter suggested a number of aims and objectives that could be implied from what respondents to the IME questionnaire saw as the reasons for teaching ethics to nurses. But what did the respondents actually state as the specific objectives of ethics teaching in courses for which they were responsible? In many cases no objectives were stated. Of the responses from general basic education, for example, all suggested that ethics was part of the curriculum, but 36% offered no specific objectives. The reasons for this fell into two main categories:

1. that this part of the curriculum had no specific objectives;
2. that because ethics was integrated throughout the curriculum no specific objectives could be identified.

This absence of objectives may be reflected in the fact that none of these respondents stated that they were able to assess students in ethics. There was, moreover, a marked contrast between responses about ethics and about other aspects of the curriculum: 12% of education centres included information about the latter, in which the learning objectives were clearly stated in behavioural terms. But in relation to ethics, even where objectives were stated, clear statements of objectives were much rarer.

In addition, many respondents from areas other than basic education did not state their objectives for ethics teaching. In post-basic education, for example, from which 16% of respondents said that the study of ethics was not part of their curriculum, a further 27% stated that it was assumed as part of the hidden curriculum; and from midwifery, more respondents (22%) did not state objectives than said that they were not teaching ethics at all. This was in contrast to responses from centres involved in community education, 98% of which were able to state objectives for their courses, and responses from different parts of the United Kingdom also varied considerably, those from Scotland and Northern Ireland generally being more explicit in this respect.

Where respondents did not state objectives for ethics teaching, however, it may have been that these were not easily accessible rather than that they did not exist. But in order now to gain a comprehensive but concise overview of those which were stated, it may be helpful to abstract those from basic general education and make a comparison, first with the aims and objectives summarised at the end of the last chapter and then with how far responses from other areas of nursing education reflected or diverged from these.

Beginning with the responses from *basic/general education*, the following inclusive list of representative objectives can be synthesised from those which were stated:

1. To develop greater awareness of moral dilemmas and ethical issues commonly encountered by the nurse in the care setting.
2. To develop knowledge, skills and attitudes in relation to ethical issues (e.g. organ transplant, brain death, euthanasia).
3. To enable nurses to approach ethical issues from a logical standpoint and thus enable them both to argue their point and to stand up for the patient's rights.
4. To encourage nurses to question their beliefs and attitudes about the patients in their care.
5. To prepare the student to accept accountability and responsibility in her role of registered nurse.

If this is examined, especially in the light of the aims and objectives summarised at the end of the last chapter, the objectives above can be reduced to the following categories:

A. Awareness of ethical issues in nursing.
B. Knowledge and skills of ethical and logical analysis.
C. Critical awareness of:

  1. the student's own beliefs and attitudes;
  2. appropriate attitudes towards patients.

D. Professionalism, with particular reference to:

  1. responsibility and accountability;
  2. advocacy and patients' rights.

These four categories cover much the same ground, if in less detail, as the aims and objectives summarised at the end of the previous chapter. Category D corresponds to the general professional aims and objectives, categories A and B to those related respectively to awareness and analysis of ethical issues, and category C to the general aim of encouraging students to understand their own and other people's values. Only the objective of providing information about different values is not explicitly included, but this could be implied from the second item in category C. One further observation about these basic education objectives, with special reference to categories B and C, is that less than 18% of respondents specified the acquisition of any sort of formal ethical theory or analysis of values.

Objectives stated by respondents responsible for courses in *areas other than basic/general education* also fit into these categories, albeit with varying emphasis. The following picture seems to emerge.

A. The general aim of creating an *awareness of ethical issues* related to nursing practice was a stated objective of respondents from most areas and in most cases this is referred to as awareness of moral or ethical dilemmas. The only major difference, in this context, between basic and other courses was that there tended to be more area-specific objectives for more specialised post-basic courses.

B. Objectives related to *ethical analysis* also were stated by many respondents, particularly those responsible for post-basic and continuing (including intensive therapy), health visiting and district nursing courses. Some knowledge of the basic subject matter of ethics or moral philosophy seems to be implied by such phrases as 'key ethical theories', 'concepts of ethics in nursing' (P/B), 'a sufficient philosophical knowledge base to aid ethical analysis' (Health visiting; HV), or the following (IT) more detailed objectives:

Define ethics . . . Give an ethical overview of the different philosophical standpoints with regard to moral principles, e.g. deontology, utilitarianism, existentialism.

Critically examine the ethical principles that underpin most philosophical points of view, e.g. the principle of human rights, the principle of honesty, the principle of justice and the principle of beneficence and non-maleficence.

Knowledge of such subject matter was seen, clearly, as important for *decision-making*. An objective stated by one (P/B) respondent, for example, was:

to provide opportunities for students to discuss, explore and apply ethical theories and concepts to decision-making.

Another, not dissimilar, (HV) objective was:

to facilitate the student's ability to analyse ethical dilemmas, in order to resolve them as far as possible.

A third, more specific, (IT) objective stated:

to examine ethical decision-making models and use one model to explore ethical dilemmas.

A further aspect of objectives concerned with ethical analysis was the expansion of 'define ethics' by the following (IT):

Explore the relationship between legal constraints, social obligations or expectations and ethical decisions.

This analytical or critical approach, however, was not always the context envisaged for the study of these issues, as can be seen by considering objectives that (omitting C for the moment) come under the next heading.

D. *Professional* rather than analytical objectives were most often stated by midwifery respondents. One (M) variant of the objective stated in the previous paragraph was:

to make students aware of professional and statutory information about ethics and professional care.

'Ethics' here, presumably, was being used with 'professional ethics' rather than 'moral philosophy' in mind. A similarly more prescriptive or normative approach to ethics is implied by the following (M) responses, stating as objectives:

to make students aware of mothers' and partners' rights towards their own health care duiring pregnancy;
the ability to promote and safeguard the well-being and interests of women and their families;
to improve the quality of care of mothers, partners and families, by being aware of ethical issues.

The last of these objectives came from a list, which, if stated in full, may help to bring out the professional rather than analytical orientation of these midwifery responses. It reads:

The student will have:
1. further development of the awareness of professional responsibility and accountability;
2. a deep understanding of the need to maintain confidentiality;
3. an awareness of the customs, values and beliefs of the women and their families, and show regard for the same;
4. the ability to promote and safeguard the well-being and interests of women and their families;
5. an understanding of the ethical constraints that may be involved in research studies.

C. The third objective in the above list overlaps with the category concerned with *values*, in particular with the values of other people. The relationship between these and the student's own values was stated by another (M) respondent in the following terms:

> To help the students look widely and understand other views and help them reach their own standards within which they can live and work, and at the same time look after women and their families without imposing their own standards (e.g. not believing in abortion but supporting a family who decide that abortion is right for them).

A further (M) respondent put this more concisely as:

> To help students identify their own ethical views and consider how these influence their professional attitudes.

A not dissimilar objective was implied by the (IT) respondent who stated:

> To enable individuals to examine personal/professional/political values and beliefs in relation to nursing practice.

One way of complementing this objective was referred to by respondents from mental and mental handicap nursing who, more commonly than in other areas, reported that their programmes included some form of attitude or value-clarification exercise.

2. SUMMARY OF OBJECTIVES

The variety of objectives specifically stated in responses to the IME questionnaire confirms the impression that ethics is being taught to nurses for aims that, in practice, may be difficult to combine. There seems to be general agreement on the desirability of the objectives summarised as category A – to increase the awareness of ethical issues in nursing – but it is not clear how much agreement there is on the specific content of categories B, C and D or whether or not these are compatible with each other.

Most difficult to render compatible are the objectives of D with those of B and C. The former seek to educate nurses as responsible and accountable professionals, with emphasis on the nursing profession's particular responsibility for advocacy and defending the rights of patients. The objectives of D are thus normative and even prescriptive; that is, they are concerned with commending particular attitudes and forms of behaviour to nurses. Against these objectives, however, those of B and C are critical and analytical: they are concerned with asking individuals to question their own and other people's moral views and values. But in doing this, of course, the attitudes and forms of behaviour commended by the objectives of D cannot escape critical scrutiny either.

These normative and critical objectives, however, may not be as incompatible with one another as appears at first sight. As already suggested, 'to commend the profession's own standards of conduct, competence and caring' is a proper objective of all nursing education. But ethics teaching in particular provides an opportunity for critical examination and questioning of those standards, in the hope that the reasons why the profession has adopted them may become clearer. At this point, it may be appropriate to say a little more about the reasons for entertaining this hope.

Nursing education properly seeks to commend attitudes and forms of behaviour which serve the goals of the profession. But a major professional goal of nursing is to provide individualised care, and a critical factor is the individuality not only of the person cared for but also of the carer. Thus the effectiveness of nursing care depends not only on the competent performance of caring functions but also on whether the nurse *cares* for the patient sufficiently for there to be some degree of openness or reciprocity in their relationship.

The main limitation on reciprocity in this relationship, clearly, is the nurse's need to continue functioning in a professional capacity relative to the patient's degree of dependency. But how much reciprocity each nurse finds compatible with functioning professionally will depend, in turn, on his or her individual professional development. If (to take the extreme case) the nurse's attitudes and behaviour

simply represent learned or habitual conformity to external professional norms, the unpredictable demands of openness and reciprocity
may be experienced primarily as a threat to the performance of other
caring functions.

The demands of reciprocity are less likely to be experienced as a
threat, however, if the nurse, in his or her education, has internalised
the _reasons_ why the norms have been commended. In this case, the
nurse will understand that these norms are relative to the ends and
limitations of nursing care and, because of this, will have greater
confidence in adapting the norms, when appropriate, to the demands
of reciprocity. This again is analogous to ordinary inter-personal
relationships, in which the more self-understanding one individual
has, the more able he or she is to hear what the other is saying and to
know his or her own capacities and limitations in responding to this.
With this in mind, the critical and analytical objectives of ethics
teaching (which ask individuals to question their own and other
people's moral views and values) can be seen as complementary to
commending particular professional attitudes and forms of behaviour.
Insofar as the latter _are_ commendable, the educational process of
questioning them will lead nurses, in due course, to hold and act on
them with greater confidence and effectiveness.

From the discussion so far it seems evident that the stated objectives
of teaching reported by the respondents to the IME questionnaire, if
these objectives are all taken together, cover the main areas and aspects
of ethics teaching relevant to nursing. What is not evident, however,
is that all these aspects are covered in each course where ethics is
reported to be taught. But again, since each aspect appears to be
reflected in the objectives of one course or another, it should be
possible in principle for all ethics courses or teaching to embody
objectives from the four main categories, concerned respectively with
awareness, analysis, values and professionalism.

The fact that this is not yet the case need not be seen as a matter for
discouragement or undue criticism. The teaching of ethics to nurses
appears to be developing in pace with nursing's 'emerging professional conscience'. As this emerges further the objectives of ethics teaching
may become more clear and more generally agreed. In this context,
moreover, it may be remarked that no ideal model of ethics teaching
from other disciplines or professions is available for adoption. Moral
philosophy itself, although an ancient discipline, is still in the throes of
freeing itself from a recent preoccupation with theoretical to the
exclusion of practical questions. And again medicine, the profession

closest to nursing, is no further (and perhaps less far) along than nursing in making provision for ethics teaching in medical schools.

At this stage then, while the main categories of objective for ethics teaching may be clear, the objectives themselves may still be described in a variety of different and provisional ways. With this in mind, it may be appropriate at this point to introduce the first two recommendations of the Working Party responsible for designing and commenting on the IME survey. These restate, in a different way, some of the main points made so far.

3. WORKING PARTY RECOMMENDATIONS

1. The teaching of ethics in nursing, midwifery and health visiting should be concerned with:

 a. value judgments and implicit values, as well as acute moral dilemmas;
 b. the logic of decision making in everyday practice;
 c. critical analysis of moral arguments in relation to cases;
 d. reason and emotion in ethics.

2. The objectives of ethics teaching should be stated explicitly. These should encourage:

 a. awareness of the nature of moral choice in health care;
 b. the ability to argue clearly and justify a view, giving reasons and examples;
 c. an ability to identify and discuss ethical aspects of the care of a specific patient or client;
 d. respect for the differing moral views of colleagues and patients or clients.

4. COURSES AND CONTENT

The number of courses or other forms of ethics teaching reported by respondents to the IME questionnaire will be discussed in the next chapter. In this context, however, it might be appropriate to ask what the content of the courses reported was and how far this reflects the objectives discussed above.

Two questions were asked on this subject. The first was on what topics were felt most important to clinical competence and from where it was felt that professional guidance came on such matters. There was little variation in answer to this question. A large proportion of respondents (including 47% from basic/general education and 42% from midwifery) did not answer at all. Most of those who did, especially but not only respondents from midwifery, referred to a code of conduct, notably that of the UKCC.

Where particular issues were mentioned as important these were often what could be characterised more as standard medical ethics issues rather than nursing ethics issues, for example issues of basic/general education such as abortion, euthanasia and transplantation. From post-basic education similar issues were identified but tended to be associated more closely with the specific nature of the course, for example, brain death and transplantation issues appeared more frequently in courses on high dependency nursing, and euthanasia more frequently in courses on care of the dying. Midwifery respondents also tended to mention standard medical ethics topics related to midwifery practice.

Characterising topics of this kind as 'standard medical ethics issues' may be misleading, however, since while they are of concern to doctors, they normally also involve nurses and patients or clients, and hence might properly be regarded as among the important concerns of health care ethics. Their importance for nursing ethics and clinical competence relative to other issues may thus depend on what aspects of these topics are discussed and whether or not they are studied in the context of other issues more specific to nursing ethics. In this respect, two further lists of topics reported by (B/G) respondents may be seen as broadening the context. These were:

1. Difficult choices in relation to:

   a. priorities of nursing care;
   b. high dependency care;
   c. discharge of patients into the community;
   d. allocation of resources;
   e. meeting the expectations of society, the individual patient and fellow professionals.

2. a. Patients' rights, i.e. dignity, information, freedom to choose.
   b. Data protection.
   c. Transplantation.

> d. Dilemmas of health economics, e.g. heart transplants versus
>   care of elderly patients.
> e. Drug trials, placebos, etc.

While some topics, particularly 2c, 2d and 2e, may again be characterised as 'standard medical ethics issues', their relevance to nursing ethics and clinical competence here will also depend on the aspects and context of discussion. The role of nurses in a team making decisions about transplantation could be an example of this, as would how a nurse might deal with questions from patients taking part in a randomised controlled trial. Or again, the apparently rather abstract question of 'dilemmas of health economics' may be used to open a discussion in which students begin to examine their own values in the light of their attitudes to transplants or elderly patients respectively. In this context it may be precisely by asking students to argue the case on either side of an acute moral dilemma (which may rarely be encountered in practice) that the implicit values underlying their own and others' value judgments are clarified. A similar justification may be offered for the reference in the above list (which includes more specifically nursing topics) to 'difficult choices'.

The IME questionnaire asked not only about topics considered important but also about those which were actually covered in ethics teaching. In response to this question a great variety of topics was reported. Some indication of this may be gained from Table 1, which shows the percentage of centres in which these topics were covered.

From this table it is evident that some of the topics most commonly covered were those in group c. Most of these focus on medical procedures or critical events, with special emphasis in post-basic and midwifery responses on analogous topics of special concern to these areas. The topics covered in group b, mostly less popular but still well-represented, are mainly concerned with patient-centred issues. Together with the more general topics in group c, groups a and b can be seen as belonging to a common core of health-care ethics topics. In this respect the relevance of those topics to nursing ethics will again depend on how far their nursing as well as general health-care implications are drawn out. Much the same, of course, might be said of the topics in group c, which also are of concern to other health professionals, although their inclusion in this context presumably signifies a primary interest in nursing.

The fact that many of the topics in group c were not specified as being covered by many schools or centres does not necessarily mean

Table 1. Topics covered in ethics teaching in different centres

Topic	Percentage		
	Basic	Post-basic	Midwifery
a. Abortion/TOP	98	88	100
Euthanasia	100	92	
Transplantation	97	69	
ECT	42	17 (39)★	
Screening			32
Modes of delivery			42
Invasive procedures			29
Induction of labour			98
Care of the neonate			98
Handicapped neonates	40	23	97
Death of a baby			100
Family planning			78
Health promotion			45
b. Consent to treatment			
Informed consent	74	78	45
Patient autonomy	52	43	23
Patients' rights	52	63	
Patient protection	2	9	95
Maternal *vs* foetal rights			18
Confidentiality	51	86	78
Truth-telling	17	18	
Risk-taking	2★★	4★★	
c. Professionalism	64	74	
Code of Conduct			16
Accountability/Responsibility	48	56	88
Patient advocacy	68	56	
Quality assurance	19	21	
Interprofessional relationships	28	34	
Research ethics	2	8	46
d. Communication			56
Ethico-legal issues	35	45	
Religious/racial issues			12
Resources	15	33	

★ Courses in RMN training   ★★ Courses in Mental Handicap

that they are not studied or discussed, for example, as aspects of the most popular topics in group a or the more patient-centred topics in group b. Once again, much will depend on how these topics are taught and also by whom, matters that will be discussed in the next chapter. To conclude this chapter, however, it may be observed that stories (or cases) and people (or patients) are of greater general interest than concepts and codes, and that the most influential teachers of ethics, both religious and secular, have often used stories and people as the initial focus of their teaching, from which they have proceeded to draw out its more general and deeper meanings. A similar procedure may well justify the popularity of the topics in groups a and b, particularly if the topics listed under c and d are used as a check-list of aspects that should not be left out of the discussion.

4 | Teaching and Assessment

1. COURSES AND TEACHING TIME

The course objectives and content discussed in the previous chapter were those of courses actually being undertaken. But in what proportion of centres do such courses exist? And of what kind and amount of teaching do they consist?

Ethics appears to be taught universally in basic education. The IME survey received replies from 77% of centres with basic education programmes of all kinds (see Appendix I) and almost 100% of these stated that the study of ethics was part of their curriculum. The very small percentage (1.4%) of respondents who said that ethics was not part of their curriculum indicated that it would be included when the curriculum was reviewed in the near future. (This, presumably, was of necessity, since new National Board recommendations state that ethics should be part of any new curriculum submitted for validation.)

In responses from post-basic education (which are difficult to analyse, for reasons stated in Appendix I), there appears to be less ethics teaching than in basic education: as mentioned in the previous chapter about 16% of respondents said that the study of ethics was not part of the curriculum for which they had responsibility, while 27% said that it was part of the hidden curriculum. Of the 26 centres with post-basic courses in intensive therapy nursing, 11 replied that ethics was taught. In basic midwifery programmes 24% of respondents stated that the study of ethics was not included, many adding that because it was not compulsory there was no time for it at present. But again, 50% of respondents added that they believed that ethics was going to be made statutory and that they intended to include it in the syllabus in the near future and certainly before the next validation visit.

In contrast with post-basic and midwifery courses, all community education programmes reported courses in ethics. In 76% of centres replying these were integrated courses, and in 24% both integrated and separate courses. In basic education, also, a high proportion (80%) of ethics courses were integrated and a similar pattern was reported from post-basic courses and midwifery: in the latter, 83% of the 66% of courses offering a formal course in ethics stated that this was integrated. The 11 intensive care centres with ethics courses reported both integrated and separate types.

The high proportion of integrated courses makes it difficult to form a clear overall picture of the amount of ethics teaching actually being undertaken. Responses from basic education, for example, generally gave the impression that the universal study of ethics refers to the discussion of ethical issues, and while 80% of courses are integrated throughout the curriculum according to subject area, the precise method of integration was often poorly described. It mostly seemed to be informal in nature, relying on tutors and students to raise a particular issue at an appropriate time. No timings, moreover, were available for the integrated courses and their structure was commonly described in such terms as 'a thread that begins in the foundation course and runs through the programme'. A similar difficulty arises in interpreting the post-basic, integrated courses, and the number of hours devoted to ethics in midwifery integrated courses could, again, often not be identified specifically. Two (M) responses illustrate the difficulty:

> Ethical considerations are discussed with each part of the curriculum to which they are appropriate, i.e. those with ethical implications. Ethics is not a separate part of the curriculum.

> [Ethics] is not laid down and taught as a formal subject, but it is discussed as the occasion arises.

If those centres that did give times can be taken as typical, the average period devoted to the discussion of ethics within the 18-month midwifery training course is 3 hours. A similar number of hours was reported from other areas.

In post-basic education the shorter certified courses and the continuing education programmes usually held a single 2- to 3-hour session for the discussion of ethical issues related to their particular area of study.

In intensive care courses discussion took the form of a study day or period, usually in the middle of the 6 months, with an average of 4 hours, and a range from 1 to 8, devoted to ethics. Further ethical discussion was integrated throughout the course as particular topics came up. In the separate education programmes the average duration of ethics teaching was 2.5 hours, with a range from 1 to 6 hours.

In basic education most (74%) of the 18 centres offering separate as well as integrated ethics teaching devoted about 4 hours or less to this and only two had more than 10 hours scheduled. Most of the separate teaching took place as part of the introductory block of nurse training, with this teaching being consolidated in the final block at the end of training. Ethics teaching in degree courses, by contrast, was often more ambitious. Of the 22 undergraduate and postgraduate courses reported, 17 had separate courses of between 10 and 20 hours.

2. INTEGRATED AND OTHER TEACHING

A high proportion of ethics teaching in nursing, midwifery and health visiting appears to be integrated with other teaching. This is particularly appropriate for those aspects of ethics teaching with normative or professional objectives, which are the familiar and proper concern of all nursing education. It is also appropriate that the critical study of nursing ethics should be grounded in the practical and scientific aspects of nursing. Aristotle, one of the first great systematisers of ethics, argued that it was not an exact science but one which had to be content with broad conclusions, since its aim was 'not *knowing* but *doing*'. Many of the reasons why ethics is seen as important for nursing education would clearly be disregarded if it were taught purely as an academic subject divorced from practice. It is unlikely that such a theoretical study would be popular with students.

Integrated courses, on the other hand, do have one obvious disadvantage. This is reflected in the responses to the IME questionnaire, which stated that it was not always possible to identify what was being taught about ethics or where it was being done. This difficulty was greatest, presumably, in courses (for example, some continuing education programmes) that have negotiated curricula and vary greatly from group to group. To overcome this difficulty it may be useful for tutors to have a check-list of the kinds of topic and objective mentioned in the previous chapter. With this in mind, a variety of examples and arguments relevant to the subject matter of any particular integrated course could be prepared in advance and introduced as time and opportunity allow (using the 'Socratic' approach outlined in section 4 of chapter 2). An approach of this kind makes it more likely that the tutors will find time and opportunity to discuss issues on which they have taken time and trouble to prepare material.

An approach of this kind begins from a point at which students' interests are engaged and involves them as much as possible in discussion as the argument develops. The most effective ethics teacher, in fact, may be the one whose main contribution is to ask the most appropriate leading questions at the optimal times, thus holding the ring, so that the focus of the discussion remains on ethical rather than other kinds of argument, and counter-examples most relevant to the topic are considered in the time available. The main qualifications for this are the tutor's own educational grounding in ethical argument and the development of this through a lively interest in the ethical aspects of everyday nursing practice. The point here is not that every tutor should be a moral philosopher, which would be as undesirable as it is impractical, but that tutors should be sufficiently ahead of the students in their knowledge of ethics to feel confident about leading the discussion. More will be said below about the training of teachers, but at this point it may be sufficient to observe that the minimum required by them is no more than can be found in any basic ethics textbook, together with some awareness of educational group dynamics.

Given the appropriately prepared teachers, then, integrated courses may well be able to cover much of the necessary ground of nursing ethics. However, there is also a strong case for some teaching time to be set aside specifically for ethics teaching, particularly in basic education but also, until that is achieved, in other courses. If, at an early stage in their education, students learn something about the background and language of ethics, they are likely to discuss ethical issues that arise later more comfortably and constructively. An introduction of this kind, for example, could help students to understand the difference between normative and critical ethics, so that ethics is seen as a matter not only of professional 'do's' and 'don'ts' but also of moral argument and of questioning received opinions and practices. In this context something could be said about roles, rules and relationships, decision-making and the different theories, principles and approaches of ethics.

Such an introduction to ethics need and should not be of a highly abstract kind. The theoretical grid which ethics superimposes upon everyday experience is never more than a tentative attempt at mapping out moral understanding; moral intuitions and decision-making skills are learnt in many places other than the classroom. The significance of ethical theory is thus best brought out by beginning as far as possible from everyday examples concerned with value judgments as well as moral dilemmas.

3. TEACHING METHODS AND AIDS

What teaching methods and aids are being used to help nursing students learn about ethics? The most popular methods, clearly, are those described as discussion and debate. 'Discussion' was mentioned by 95% of respondents from basic education and 87% from midwifery, 'debate' by 65% of the former and 42% of the latter. 'Discussion' and 'debate' together were mentioned by 89% of post-basic education respondents. These methods also appeared to be favoured in other areas, as was role play, which appeared in 18% of responses from basic education, 26% from midwifery and 30% from intensive therapy courses. Most respondents (including 82% from basic education) reported using a mixture of methods.

Formal lectures appear to be among the least-favoured methods of teaching ethics. In basic education they were mentioned by less than 25% of respondents, mostly as part of the introductory course of those institutions that said that they were running a separate course in ethics. A further method, reported particularly from post-basic curricula, was the use of project work and the extended essay in the teaching of ethics. In most of the responses that spoke of this in any detail it seemed that selection of an ethics-related topic in this area was optional, reflecting the personal interests of the students. In only 2 of the 67 courses reporting this kind of work was an ethics topic compulsory.

The main teaching aids used in ethics teaching appear to be books, journal articles and videos. Respondents from both basic and midwifery education reported using television documentary recordings. Many basic education tutors, however, complained of a lack of useful video material, which they felt would be particularly appropriate for this type of teaching. Midwifery tutors also complained of a general shortage of relevant teaching material on ethics in midwifery, and about 37% of midwifery respondents stated that they used no additional teaching material at all. Some schools engaged in basic education provided extensive reading lists, containing a wide variety of books, both British and American, as well as journal articles. A full list of these as well as of midwifery educational material is given in the bibliography.

4. DISCUSSION

The teaching methods and aids reported make it clear that some kind of discussion method is generally seen as the best way of studying ethical issues in nursing education. The various teaching materials mentioned would all appear to be ways of stimulating discussion, and 'debate' is normally a differently structured version of the same method. In some respects, of course, 'debate' may have advantages over 'discussion' for ethics teaching, since a good debate forces participants to think through the position they have to defend or attack. Role-play, similarly, helps those involved to realise the emotional aspects of moral arguments with which they may not identify personally. Greater use of this method in intensive therapy courses than elsewhere was significantly linked with sessions dealing with communication between professionals, and role-play in general is a useful way of exploring areas where the interests of ethics and communication overlap.

The limited use of lectures as a teaching method may be related to the extent to which ethics is taught in integrated courses, but it may also reflect the popular prejudice that ethics is simply a matter of opinion. While this view is not without a grain of truth, in the sense that all ethical arguments are contestable, it glosses over the fact that some ethical arguments are better than others in terms of their consistency, coherence and correspondence with ascertainable facts. A considerable body of knowledge exists in this area, and also with respect to logical argument, which is helpful in avoiding many common fallacies in ethics, such as rhetorical or circular arguments, unjustified generalisations and vague or ambiguous reasoning. The quality of moral reasoning and logical argument employed by different people may, in practice, be highly variable, and some knowledge of these aspects of ethics and logic can promote thinking which is both clearer and more communicable to others.

How far lectures are the best method of communicating this body of knowledge is debatable. The main advantage of a lecture is that it allows the development of a sustained argument so that its force may be more fully felt. But in practice, of course, whether or not it *is* felt may depend on qualities in the lecturer that catch the interest of and evoke a response from the audience. While some of the skills of good lecturing can be learnt, not all of the necessary qualities can be taught. In the context of ethics teaching, therefore, it would seem unwise to rely too heavily upon this method. On the other hand, lectures need not be seen exclusively in terms of the standard 45-minute academic variety, and a combination of short lectures with discussion, debate or role-play may be, in many contexts, the most effective way of stimulating or sustaining interest so that the maximum amount is learnt in the time available.

Much the same amount may be learned also through 'discussion', even without the use of other teaching aids or methods. But a major risk of this method is that it may not challenge participants to think critically and logically about their own and other participants' moral arguments. Moreover, if the discussion ends in a vague consensus or agreement to differ, the participants may leave either with their own prejudices confirmed or with the popular misconception that there is no real point in arguing about such relative questions. The most effective argument against this conclusion, perhaps, can be provided by tutors who prepare for and structure the discussion sufficiently to persuade their students that it is worth taking seriously.

5. ASSESSMENT

A different kind of argument that students may use to themselves for taking a subject seriously, of course, is whether the subject is examined or otherwise assessed. What evidence is there of ethics being taken seriously in this way in nursing education?

On this question replies to the IME questionnaire suggest some discontinuity between theory and practice. Respondents were asked how important they felt ethical competence to be to general clinical competence. The question was asked in terms of a five-point scale, and the results are displayed in Table 2.

Despite the importance thus accorded to it, however, ethical competence is not commonly assessed in nursing education. Of the responses from basic education, 132 said that students were not assessed in this subject in any way, and of the 48 respondents who said that their students were assessed, none held a formal separate examination in ethics. Responses from post-basic education were similar: the shorter certified courses and continuing education programmes did not assess ethical competence in 98% of their curricula, while

Table 2.   The importance of ethical competence to clinical competence

	Basic (%)	Post-basic (%)	Midwifery (%)	Community (%)
Essential	87	85	91	88
Very important	11	12	6	8
Important	2	3	3	4
Quite important	0	0	0	0
Not at all important	0	0	0	0

post-basic (certified) courses or those related to professional development did not assess in 88% of cases. In midwifery education, also, the
great majority of courses included no ethics assessment. Only in
degree programmes was assessment normal. Some sort of examination in ethics, constituting part of the final degree award, was included
in 95% of these.

Where there was assessment, degree courses apart, the most
common form was by essays, other written work or clinical assessment. Where this was done in basic education, respondents described
it as a way in which tutors looked for some awareness of the ethical
dimension in nursing. They rarely made explicit, however, at what
level this awareness should be, or how precisely it was evaluated. Nor
was information of this kind forthcoming from other areas of nursing
education (again, degree courses apart), and most assessment appears
to be informal.

This lack of assessment in what is considered to be such an
important area may be attributable to at least three causes. The first
would be something roughly similar to the popular prejudice about
ethics mentioned above. If ethics is simply a matter of opinion, how
can it be assessed? This view is perhaps what lay behind one (B/G)
respondent's remark that some teachers regarded ethics as a 'peripheral topic' and 'one that cannot be taught'.

A more serious difficulty in assessing ethics may relate to its place in
many integrated curricula. As another (B/G) respondent put it:

> Whilst some attempt has been made to categorise 'ethics' as a
> subject for the purpose of the questionnaire, because the curriculum
> is designed as a spiral model with self-directed learning, specific
> areas and subjects cannot be essentially identified separately. Ethics
> is integrated throughout virtually every aspect of caring – beliefs,

attitudes, opinions, feelings, rights, etc. Evaluation of achievement is primarily determined by experts and the experience of professionals (tutors, supervisors, role models within the various exposure areas). Consumers have representative roles that monitor effects.

Two kinds of difficulty appear to be expressed in this response. One concerns the problems of assessing any traditional subject within a curriculum of the kind described. The other seems to arise from identifying ethics, and hence ethics teaching, with progress towards the professional and value objectives identified in the previous chapter. Progress of this kind is clearly difficult to assess, for the reasons given by the respondent and also because those involved in assessment are themselves likely to have different views on what constitutes such progress. In this context, however, as in assessing clinical skills, the difficulty of devising scientific forms of assessment does not necessarily mean that no assessment is possible. Measurement is, after all, a means to and not the end of assessment, which is to encourage standards of excellence.

To this end, it can be suggested, self-evaluation may have something (even if not everything) to contribute. In discussing this subject members of the IME Working Party suggested that critical incident analysis or a 'hopes, fears and expectations' exercise might be useful. In the latter, where students write down their 'hopes, fears and expectations', at the beginning of one session, and at the beginning of the next write down what they have learnt, a formative self-assessment of progress may be made. It may, as one tutor pointed out, be something very simple and practical, but nevertheless very important, as in the case of one student who wrote, 'I learnt that Rastafarians don't eat pork'. Or again, as another observed:

It is surprising how often the students realise that what they were doing was simply awful; and this is a self-evaluation.

A third reason for lack of assessment in ethics teaching may simply be that ethics teaching in nursing education is still a developing area. Assessment by essays and other written work is clearly being used in a number of centres, and this method is highly appropriate for teaching concerned with awareness and analysis of ethical issues. The method is, after all, little different from assessment of ethics learning in the education of other professions and in moral philosophy courses at university, college and 'A'-level standards. While it is a new departure in nursing education and requires to be adapted to the particular needs of nursing practice, there is no reason to expect that it will not eventually become widely accepted.

6. WORKING PARTY RECOMMENDATIONS

To conclude this section, two further recommendations of the IME Working Party may be recorded.

3. To achieve the objectives of ethics teaching in nursing education, the following are necessary in any course:

a. A separate module as well as integrated teaching.
b. A series of lectures, seminars or tutorials that explore the interactions between practice, personal views and philosophical arguments.
c. Ethics teaching developing progressively through the course.
d. Teaching in small groups, wherever possible, to facilitate student participation.

4. To the same end, the following should be encouraged:

a. Formal assessment on a regular basis of how far the objectives are being achieved.
b. Research to determine the most appropriate methods of teaching and formal assessment.

7. TEACHING IN THE CLINICAL AREA

Not all teaching of ethics to nursing students would necessarily have been known to respondents to the IME questionnaire. An example of this might be some informal learning sessions in the clinical area not arranged by tutors. Members of the IME Working Party varied in their own impressions of how much teaching of this kind took place but considered that it was most likely to take place in the specialist areas. A paediatrician, for example, might set up a group of medical and nursing students to discuss ethical issues that had arisen in the care of a particular patient, and something similar might happen in the care of the elderly and other specialties. Moreover, as one member of the Working Party put it:

Certainly, in the coffee rooms of the specialist areas nurses are sitting down and trying to work out these ethical issues in their minds, and discussing them. I would say that at least once a week I get involved with staff in the Accident and Emergency department, discussing a situation that occurred that morning and what they thought about what happened; and it can get quite heated and very interesting.

The multidisciplinary learning aspects mentioned above will be discussed in the next chapter. At this point, however, it might be sufficient to say that the importance of all such informal learning sessions cannot be underestimated. A skilful teaching response to an incident in which something has been seen (or failed to be seen) to have gone wrong may make an ethical point or raise an ethical question much more tellingly than in less involving contexts. Or again, much may be learnt about an issue such as autonomy when the patient concerned, or the parents of a handicapped child for example, are involved in the discussion, or the views and values of a known patient are represented by a nurse.

A major problem about teaching ethics in the clinical area, however, is lack of time. Often, this is far too short to begin to do more than disentangle one or two of the most difficult emotional knots in or between those taking part in the discussion. Any attempt to relate the relevant threads to the wider context of ethics may well be impossible, even for the most skilful teacher. Because of this, ethics teaching in the classroom takes on an even greater significance, since it can provide time and space for students to express their feelings about their past experience and, for example, not to feel a failure if they have not handled an experience as well as they might.

Commending this aspect of classroom teaching, however, should not be seen as in any way diminishing the responsibility of nurses and others in the clinical area to encourage student learning about ethics in this context. If those in the clinical area feel that they lack the expertise of ethics teachers, it may be pointed out that effective teaching of nursing ethics cannot do without precisely the experience they possess or their mature reflection on that experience. As such teaching increasingly comes to be incorporated throughout nursing education, it may be hoped that more and more nurses will feel that they have the expertise necessary for teaching ethics at the level appropriate to their responsibilities. In the meantime, however, one practical way forward is to invite experienced clinical practitioners to take part in formal ethics teaching, where the experience of teaching may also be a learning experience that the practitioner can make use of later in the clinical area.

8. SUPPORT SYSTEMS AND CO-ORDINATION

Ethics teaching in the clinical area may well be seen to overlap with a further question addressed by the IME survey. This asked if there were any formal support systems within the relevant institution to help staff cope with ethical problems that arose in practice. In reply 88% of institutions reported no formal systems but described informal activities, including peer support, management, occupational health departments and the hospital chaplain, while about 19% of respondents said that if they had a very specific problem, they might go to the hospital ethics committee or to the District Health Authority. About 10% of those who reported no formal system added that they would like such a system to exist.

Providing support to help staff cope with ethical problems in practice is clearly not the same thing as making provision for ethics teaching in the clinical area. The counselling and the teaching skills respectively required for these purposes may differ and are often possessed by different people. Nevertheless, the objectives of counselling and management also have much in common with those of ethics teaching, since their common aim is that of learning to respond more adequately to the problems involved. Thus there may be ways in which those concerned with support and those concerned with teaching can co-operate fully.

Discussing how this might be done, the IME Working Party did not believe that it was in a position to recommend any specific support system. The needs of the different institutions, and especially different clinical areas, were too varied for this and in certain contexts may be met most appropriately by a multidisciplinary or other system. (An example is the use, suggested above, of hospital ethics committees for advice. Such committees are concerned with the ethics of research, but if, as in some cases happens, they are used for wider purposes, thought might be given to whether or not a hospital ethics committee, as such, is required.)

9. WORKING PARTY RECOMMENDATION

While not wishing to recommend a specific support system, however, the Working Party did believe that it was important to develop new and appropriate ways of helping staff and students cope with clinical ethical problems. To this end, therefore, it made the following recommendation:

5. a. Within each institution where ethical problems are encountered in the clinical area, a group should be convened to consider the most appropriate means of providing support, for students and practitioners in relation to these problems.

   b. Initiatives towards this end should be undertaken as a priority by the co-ordinator designated in Recommendation 8 (below).

In making this recommendation the Working Party was aware that the process of developing appropriate support systems was likely to be slow, and that the people best suited to serve on such groups were already likely to be serving on a variety of other groups and committees. Because of this it seemed appropriate in the first instance to encourage designated individuals, and particularly those already concerned with ethics in the context of teaching, to take an initiative. (Further information about these individuals is given in the next chapter.) As to membership of such groups, the Working Party again did not wish to make specific recommendations, but considered that they might include such individuals as a senior manager, the occupational health nurse, the hospital chaplain and a clinical psychologist, together with the clinical practitioners.

5 | Students and Teachers

1. MULTIDISCIPLINARY LEARNING: RECOMMENDATION

Many ethical issues encountered in nursing practice also are encountered by members of other health professions. How far are nursing students being prepared for this by learning about ethics in discussion with students in training for these other professions? As was mentioned in the last chapter, some such multidisciplinary learning may take place in informal contexts in various specialist areas. But does it take place in the more formal contexts reported by respondents to the IME questionnaire?

No form of multidisciplinary learning was reported by midwifery schools, nor from any general post-basic nor intensive therapy course. But it was more likely to be found in mental nursing and particularly mental handicap training, where sessions with social workers and psychologists seemed common. In community education a little under half of all institutions provided for multidisciplinary learning, although in practice this mostly involved different nursing-related groups getting together for discussions. In 27 centres, however, particularly in health visiting programmes, student social workers were also involved, and in two institutions some sessions included GP trainees. Of the 147 replies from basic education only 16 included any kind of multidisciplinary learning; where this took place the other students included medical students, dental students, clinical psychologists, health visitors and, in one case, medical photographers. In these courses about 20% to 30% of the total length of the course was spent in such mixed discussion.

Opinion of these courses reported by respondents was generally favourable, suggesting that such groups led to a more open exchange of views and a greater appreciation of other people's values. On the other hand, some teachers felt that unless the nursing students already had had a firm grounding in their professional education they could feel intimidated, especially by medical students. One teacher commented that:

> the [nursing] students often felt alienated by the views of the medical students, but felt that they could not articulate their own.

While the IME Working Party appreciated this last point, it believed that it was important for nursing students to learn to articulate their own views in multidisciplinary learning contexts. The use of multidisciplinary learning in the post-basic training of district nurses was, it was argued, a particularly good example of this, and where a case-study approach was used students in training for the different health professions could share and thrash out their differences. In sessions of this kind, however, the Working Party emphasised, skilled teachers and facilitators from the different disciplines were needed in order to ensure that students from different disciplines and with different points of view were given an adequate opportunity to express themselves. If this were done well, the students would later be able to discuss ethical issues arising in practice more constructively.

It was also noted that in some centres nursing students shared informal extra-curricular learning sessions with medical and other health-care students, through participation in the various student medical groups associated with the Institute of Medical Ethics. Multidisciplinary activities of this kind outside the curriculum were to be commended. In relation to a more formal curricular provision, the Working Party made the following recommendation:

6.   Where possible, institutions should encourage participation in multidisciplinary learning on ethical issues involving students from other disciplines.

2. MULTIDISCIPLINARY TEACHING: RECOMMENDATION

While teachers from different disciplines are needed to facilitate multidisciplinary learning, they may also have a part to play in sessions where nursing students learn on their own about ethics. From the replies to the IME questionnaire it is clear that while the majority of those teaching ethics to nursing students are themselves nurses, a variety of other disciplines and professions also are involved in the teaching.

Among the other professions involved doctors did not play a large role. In basic education, for example, they took part in programmes in only 24 schools, and in these cases were mainly paediatricians specialising in neonatology. On midwifery courses paediatricians and obstetricians were the most common teachers other than midwives, but were selected to teach on the basis of their medical expertise rather than any particular expertise in ethics. (Only 16% of midwifery teaching centres, in fact, reported sessions devoted to ethics and the guest medical lecturer normally also had to be able to talk about a variety of other topics.) A similar pattern of specialist guest medical lectures seemed to obtain in post-basic courses, although medical staff were largely absent from community education courses.

Other professionals involved included judges, Home Office representatives and drug squad personnel, all in mental nursing courses; and in intensive care courses, transplant co-ordinators and specialist social workers. Again, many of the sessions in which these individuals were involved were not exclusively devoted to ethics, but a discussion of ethics was expected to arise as part of a general topic. In community education (the training courses for which all take place in Institutes of Higher Education) lecturers from other disciplines were involved in teaching and included health education lecturers, developmental psychologists, health and social policy lecturers and counsellors.

Philosophers, while commonly teaching ethics on degree courses, were not well represented in other areas. In basic education, for example, only 12 centres had a guest lecturer with a formal philosophical training. These lecturers taught mainly in schools that offered a separate course in ethics as part of the introductory block. The philosophy teachers were normally invited because they were known to a member of the tutorial staff, who often had attended a course run by them.

The guest lecturers most commonly involved, however, were hospital chaplains. Chaplains were reported as teaching ethics in 58% of basic education programmes, 68% of midwifery courses and 67% of those post-basic (certified) courses and 89% of those continuing education courses which listed ethics as part of a stated curriculum. Chaplains were largely absent from community education programmes, however, and were less prominent in courses in Northern Ireland, where there is a more formalised structure of ethics teaching.

Reflecting on these findings, the IME Working Party considered that while guest lecturers could make a useful contribution on medical, legal, religious and other issues of importance to nursing practice, they should not be seen as a substitute for teachers of nursing ethics. Hospital chaplains, for example, often had a great deal to teach about counselling or about religious customs, values and beliefs, all of which might be related to ethical issues. Increasingly, moreover, the general and theological education of chaplains is likely to have included teaching on the ethics of health care. But this is not necessarily the case, nor can it be assumed that medical staff or members of other professions have any special expertise in discussing ethical issues. Nor, again, can it be assumed that philosophers, even those who specialise in ethics, are the most appropriate teachers of ethics to nursing students. In the case of philosophers the problem is not lack of expertise in teaching ethics but the possibility that they lack that practical experience of health-care practice necessary to ground their teaching in clinical reality and thus commend it to their students.

In the case of all such guest lecturers, then, the Working Party wished to sound a note of caution and to encourage a discriminating approach, taking account less of the office than of the expertise and experience of those to be invited. To this end it made the following recommendation:

7.   Teachers from disciplines or professions other than nursing, while often having a useful contribution to make to the teaching of nursing ethics, should not be seen as a substitute for such teaching by nursing teachers.

3. TEACHING STAFF, TRAINING AND CO-ORDINATION: RECOMMENDATION

This last recommendation appears, in fact, to be reflected in the majority of basic education programmes: from 62% of those responding it was reported that nurse tutors were the main teachers of ethics. Nurses involved in ethics teaching were not always those responsible for the course concerned. In both basic and post-basic courses specialist nursing staff were drawn upon where appropriate (for example, in 12% of basic courses, hospice staff were brought in to deal with issues related to care of the dying), and while the majority (60%) of those involved in teaching ethics to midwifery students were midwives, almost 20% of these were either still practising midwives or midwifery service managers.

How far were these nursing teachers also trained or prepared to teach ethics? Responses from other areas did not differ significantly from those for basic education where, in general, there was no formal training or preparation of the staff involved in ethics teaching. The integrated curriculum means that teachers with special training do not necessarily have any particular responsibility for the ethics component in the curriculum. By the same token, it appears that many teachers who feel comfortable with the subject may be involved in teaching it: certainly about half of the respondents from basic education included some comment by tutors expressing unease about their ability to handle ethics in the curriculum.

On the other hand, about 30% of the replies from basic education stated that one or more of their teachers had had some basic philosophical training as part of their undergraduate studies. In some 54% of the schools one or more of the tutors had attended study days where ethics, especially ethico–legal issues, had been discussed, and 10 tutors in various parts of the country were reported to be studying for one of the Master's Degrees in health care ethics or philosophy. Nevertheless, from the majority of replies it seemed that 'personal reading' or 'nothing specific' were the most commonly expressed methods of preparing nursing teachers to teach ethics. It is not surprising, therefore, as one respondent put it, that:

> teachers appear a little hesitant to move into this area, which may reflect the lack of teacher preparation.

Reviewing these responses, the IME Working Party acknowledged that because nursing ethics is still a developing subject, there is bound to be both a variety of views about what it comprises and some hesitancy among tutors about their own ability to teach it. The Working Party was anxious, moreover, as one of its members put it:

> not to discourage the amateur from getting involved in teaching ethics: he must not become so worried about not being able to do it correctly that he does not dare attempt to do it at all.

In this respect, as other members observed, it would be disastrous if ethics came to be seen as too specialised 'as in the case of some research, like some hot-house plant for those in the universities', and it was thus not seen as 'part of the trained nurse's duty in teaching the next generation'. It was important to stress, as one member of the Working Party pointed out, that 'you don't need to know everything in order to do something'.

Nevertheless, as the same member went on to remark, 'when you are getting out of your depth and need to learn more, you do need to know where to look for further help'. The Working Party agreed with this and for this reason hoped that nurses concerned with ethics teaching would themselves create the opportunities for exchanging information on a national or more local basis. (The RCN Education Association, it was suggested, was beginning to provide one such forum.) The Working Party also hoped, in this context, that more nursing teachers would take advantage of the various health care ethics courses now available; information on these is included in Appendix II.

Beyond expressing these hopes, however, the Working Party recognised a particular need for some appropriate means of developing ethics teaching and helping teachers prepare for this in particular institutions. It did not consider that this need would be best met by appointing particular members of staff as ethics teachers since this was likely to lead to over-specialisation and the feeling among other teachers that because someone else was responsible for ethics teaching, they themselves were not. A better alternative would be, in the words of the Working Party's final recommendation, the following:

8.   Each institution should designate at least one member of staff as available and responsible for co-ordinating ethics teaching in the curriculum.

In making this recommendation, the Working Party believed that both the all-pervasive and the developing aspects of ethics teaching justified (as was not necessarily justified in relation to many other subjects) an appointment of the kind recommended. Given the obvious dangers of ethics teaching being exploited by those with partisan interests, it would be important for the individual or individuals designated to be seen to be impartial or to represent a fair balance of interests. The person or persons designated would be responsible for reviewing existing teaching to discover areas that required further attention, for learning about developments in other centres that could usefully be adapted to the institutions's curriculum, and for co-ordinating the contribution of members of staff and any visiting teachers to ensure a good coverage of both practical and ethical issues. A further role for the co-ordinator has already been discussed in connection with recommendation 5 above.

4. CONCLUSION

In reviewing responses to the IME questionnaire the Working Party heard of some tutors who considered that ethics was a 'peripheral' topic, others who believed that it 'could not be taught' and others again who would have agreed with the remark:

It would be helpful to look at the current issues and problems both locally and nationally, but there just isn't time.

Such responses were less typical, however, than those which made comments such as:

Current television and media articles highlight topical areas of interest. It would be useful to know how to teach ethical principles or philosophy. Difficult to know in our situation.

Or again:

I would welcome any advice, information or results of your survey once completed.

From responses of this kind, it is evident that the teaching of ethics to nurses is an area in which there is now growing interest and considerable potential. The Working Party hopes, therefore, that the contribution of this report, however limited the scope of a single year's study, will add further stimulus to the development of a subject in which (to quote a representative response) 'the relatively recent innovation of timetabled sessions is very much appreciated by the students'.

List of Recommendations

The Working Party recommended that:

1. The teaching of ethics in nursing, midwifery and health visiting should be concerned with:

    a. value judgments and implicit values, as well as acute moral dilemmas;

    b. the logic of decision-making in everyday practice;

    c. critical analysis of moral arguments in relation to cases;

    d. reason and emotion in ethics.

2. The objectives of ethics teaching should be stated explicitly. These should encourage:

    a. awareness of the nature of moral choice in health care;

    b. the ability to argue clearly and justify a view, giving reasons and examples;

    c. an ability to identify and discuss ethical aspects of the care of a specific patient or client;

    d. respect for the differing moral views of colleagues and patients or clients.

3. To achieve the objectives of ethics teaching in nursing education, the following are necessary in any course:

    a. A separate module as well as integrated teaching.

    b. A series of lectures, seminars and tutorials that explore the interactions between practice, personal views and philosophical arguments.

    c. Ethics teaching developing progressively through the course.

    d. Teaching in small groups, wherever possible, to facilitate student participation.

4. To the same end, the following should be encouraged:

a. Formal assessment on a regular basis of how far the objectives are being achieved.

b. Research to determine the most appropriate methods of teaching and formal assessment.

5. a. Within each institution where ethical problems are encountered in the clinical area, a group should be convened to consider the most appropriate means of providing support for students and practitioners in relation to these problems.

b. Initiatives towards this end should be undertaken as a priority by the co-ordinator designated in recommendation 8 (below).

6. Where possible, institutions should encourage participation in multidisciplinary learning on ethical issues involving students from other disciplines.

7. Teachers from disciplines or professions other than nursing, while often having a useful contribution to make to the teaching of medical ethics, should not be seen as a substitute for such teaching by nursing teachers.

8. Each institution should designate at least one member of staff as available and responsible for co-ordinating ethics teaching in the curriculum.

Appendix I
Methodology
and Results

A study of the teaching of ethics in Nursing, Midwifery and Health Visiting

Methodology
The purposes of the study were to:

I (a) describe and define the nature of ethics in nursing, midwifery and health visiting

II (a) review the literature with regard to the study of ethics in nursing

 (b) investigate curricular arrangements for teaching ethics in the UK

III (a) discuss the advantages and disadvantages of different current initiatives in the teaching of ethics in nursing; to compare existing and possible developments; and to consider future directions

 (b) produce a well-documented report, making recommendations on ethics teaching addressed to those responsible for the education of nurses, midwives and health visitors.

In order to achieve the purposes stated above, a working party was convened which designed the research protocol, decided on the significance of the results obtained and produced the recommendations.

The Working Party decided that the research study should be as broad as possible and that a postal questionnaire was the most appropriate method of achieving that aim. The whole of the United Kingdom was to be surveyed and the addresses of the education centres were obtained from the appropriate National Boards.

The Working Party also wished that the various levels and types of education should be explored and therefore separate questionnaires were designed for basic, post-basic and continuing education programmes.

The responsibility for nurse education is disparate and so in an attempt to ensure that the most appropriate person completed the questionnaire, it was decided to send the basic and post-basic questionnaires to the respective Directors of Nurse/Midwifery Education and that the continuing education questionnaire should be sent to the Chief/District Nurse Officer/Advisor.

An accompanying letter explained the aims of the project and asked that the questionnaire be completed by the person most responsible for ethics education within the institution.

The questionnaires were designed by the research team in consultation with the pilot group of the Working Party. Due to the fact that there was little existing work in this field it was decided that the questions had to be open-ended in design, in the hope that the maximum amount of information could be obtained. This also meant that the analysis framework for the questionnaires had to be constructed after the pilot period. (Piloting was done in five centres of nurse education representative of all of the different types of courses being surveyed.) Computer analysis proved to be impracticable and the data had to be analysed manually using a coding and card system.

KEY (to be used in all tables of results)

B   BASIC GENERAL EDUCATION
PB   POST-BASIC (certified)
C   CONTINUING EDUCATION
M   MIDWIFERY
M(C)   MIDWIFERY (CONTINUING)
CE   COMMUNITY EDUCATION
UC   UNDERGRADUATE COURSES

RESULTS OF QUESTIONNAIRE

Tables 1 and 2 show the final response rates to the questionnaires at the end of the four month data collection period. The relatively poor responses from continuing education seemed to be a consequence of

Table 1
QUESTIONNAIRE RESPONSE RATES **(England and Wales)**

	Number sent	Number returned	% response
Basic General Education	187	147	77
Post-Basic (certified)	187	151	80
Continuing	156	64	41
Midwifery – Basic	147	124	84
– Continuing	147	98	67
Community education	85	53	62
Undergraduate courses	17	17	100

Table 2
QUESTIONNAIRE RESPONSE RATES
(Scotland and Northern Ireland)

	Number sent	Number returned	% response
Basic General Education	25	19	76
Post-Basic (certified)	25	21	84
Continuing	25	15	60
Midwifery – Basic	17	13	76
– Continuing	17	9	53
Community education	9	7	78

sending the questionnaires to Chief Nurses, who were not always able to forward them to the correct people, or they just got lost in the bureaucracy of the organisation. Some centres photocopied the questionnaire and returned separate responses for the range of courses, and although the results of these appear at the appropriate point later they only counted as one-centre responses in terms of response rates.

The results will now be discussed in question order.

Question 1
This asked the respondent to list the courses taught in their institution.

Question 2
Do you consider that the study of ethics should be part of any nursing curriculum for which you have responsibility? Please give reasons for your view.

	Yes	% No	Blank
B	98	2	0
PB	91	3	6
C	76	13	11
M	96	2	2
M(C)	99	0	1
CE	100		
UG	100		

The following reasons were most commonly mentioned for studying ethics

Reasons (%)	Type of Course						
	B	PB	C	M	M(C)	CE	UG
Professional necessity	56	76	65	87	95	92	97
Values awareness	34	34	21	56	45	47	78
Moral consideration	29	23	16	54	34	14	34
Humanitarian reasons	41	56	66	71	32	65	56

Question 3
Is the study of ethics part of your curriculum? If it is not included, please indicate why not.

Again, almost 100% replied that they seemed to be referring to ethical issues rather than ethics per se. The very small percentage of respondents who said that ethics was not currently part of their curriculum indicated that it was to be included when they rewrote their curricula in the near future. This response was not surprising in the light of the new National Board regulations about including ethics in any new curriculum before it could be validated.

Type of course	Response (%)		
	Yes	No	Blank
B	97	2	1
PB	89	4	7
C	79	11	10
M	95	4	0
M(C)	99		1
CE	100		
UG	100		

The failure to include ethics especially in post-basic and continuing education was said to be due to a shortage of time in the crowded curricula.

Question 4
What are the objectives of this part of the curriculum?

This question produced a variety of responses. Many were very brief and spoke of highlighting these issues, others were more detailed and listed a range of skills/abilities to be learnt. A more detailed analysis of these and their implications is covered in the main text, however a number of points should be mentioned at this time.

Less than 18% of total respondents (there was no significant difference between different courses in this area, with the exception of the undergraduate schemes) mentioned the acquisition of any sort of formal ethical theory of analysis of values.

36% (n = 53) of the questionnaires contained no specific response to this question. The reasons for this fell into two main categories: a) that this part of the curriculum had no specific objectives, or b) because ethics was integrated throughout the curriculum no specific objectives could be identified.

Question 5
Is the subject integrated throughout the curriculum or is it a separate course/module or both?

Type of training	Type of course (%)		
	Separate	Integrated	Both
B	4	82	14
PB	25	45	30
C	16	67	17
M	6	78	16
M(C)	34	28	48
CE	42	23	35
UG	14	8	78

The precise method of integration was poorly described and often seemed to be related to a spiral form of curriculum design. It also seemed to be quite informal in nature, i.e. it relied on the students or tutors to bring up issues at an appropriate time in the curriculum.

Question 6
If a separate course, please indicate
a) At what point in the course does it occur?
b) How much time is allocated to this subject?

Again there was a level of consistency in the answers to this question across the types of training. 64% of the distinct courses offered it initially in the introductory block, with 74% then being further consolidated during a 'management/professionalism' block somewhere near the completion of training. The remaining 36% of courses also occurred in the last third of training.

Type of course	Time allotted (hours)			
	0–4	**4–6**	**6–10**	**10+**
B	74	14	6	6
PB	78	15	7	0
C	88	10	2	0
M	46	32	18	4
M(C)	92	4	3	1
CE	64	12	14	10
UG	0	6	36	58

Question 7
If ethics is integrated throughout the curriculum, please indicate how this is achieved.

This question generally illicited a poor response. It was usually said that the discussion of ethical issues was implicit in all areas of the course. It seemed to be expected that students would raise these questions at an appropriate part in each module. The discussion of ethical issues was most commonly described as a 'thread that begins in the foundation course and is developed throughout the programme'.

Question 8
Please indicate the specialties and disciplines of the staff involved in the teaching.

Disciplines of those involved in ethics teaching							
% of courses involved							
	B	PB	C	M	M(C)	CE	UG
Nurse tutors	100	100	100	100	100	100	100
Specialist staff	43	67	72	56	74	46	23
Medical staff	12	9	27	13	5	4	18★
Philosopher	6	11	8	18	6	32	86
Police	4★★	6★★					
Judges	2★★						
Chaplain	56	47	16	47	21	11	5

★ *Only in multidisciplinary teaching (see question 10)*
★★ *In RNM courses only.*

Question 9
a) *Please indicate any specific ways in which the staff of the institution have been prepared to deal with and teach about these issues, including any ethics courses that they have attended.*

There was little formal preparation of staff: 96% of schools reported no formal preparation of their staff. However about 30% of tutors responsible for ethics teaching said that they had had some formal philosophical training as part of their own studies. About 54% of tutors said that they had attended courses where ethical or ethico–legal issues had been a major part of the programme.

b) *In the case of visiting teachers, could you explain on what basis they were chosen.*

Visiting teachers were usually selected on the basis of personal knowledge and recommendation, either for their knowledge, specific background or objectivity. Medical staff, however, seem to be selected purely on the basis of the post that they held.

Question 10

a) Are students from other disciplines taught ethics with nurses/midwives/health visitors?

b) If 'yes', which disciplines are these?

Multidisciplinary teaching is largely confined to centres of higher education where students from other disciplines are also studying. Therefore only 16 basic courses had multidisciplinary teaching sessions; these were schools attached to major hospitals where other paramedical workers were also being trained. Other students involved included medical/dental students, clinical psychologists, social workers, health visitors and in one case medical photographers.

c) What proportion of total time that the nurses/midwives/ health visitors spend in ethical discussion are they with students of other disciplines?

No respondent said that the students spent all of their time with students of other disciplines. It was felt important that the nurses had some time for isolated teaching. In general multidisciplinary teaching only occurred after some background had been given to the students. The courses usually involved 20–30% of the total time in multidisciplinary discussion.

d) Are there any obvious benefits or advantages?

The general opinion was favourable although little formal evaluation has taken place. Such groups are felt to produce more open discussion and a greater appreciation of other points of view. However, some teachers felt that unless the students had a strong grounding in the basics they could feel intimidated especially by medical students.

Question 11
a) *Are the nursing/midwifery/health visiting students assessed in this subject?*
b) *If so, how?*

Course	Type of assessment (%)			
	None	Essay	Clinical	Project
B	78	7	11	4
PB	67	12	7	14
C	84	4	6	6
M	84	5	7	4
M(C)	92	4	4	
CE	74	14	6	6
UG	0	78	14	4

Only the undergraduate courses reported having examinations in just ethics.

Question 12
Please indicate how important you consider an understanding of ethical issues to be to a nurse's/midwife's/health visitor's general professional competence.

	B	PB	C	M	M(C)	CE	UG
Essential	87	90	67	92	94	97	100
Very important	11	7	19	7	4	3	
Important	2	3	14	1	2		
Quite important							
Not at all important							

Question 13
In your curriculum what ethics topics/issues do you deal with?

Table 1. Topics covered in ethics teaching in different centres

Topic	Percentage		
	Basic	Post-basic	Midwifery
a. Abortion/TOP	98	88	100
Euthanasia	100	92	
Transplantation	97	69	
ECT	42	17 (39)★	
Screening			32
Modes of delivery			42
Invasive procedures			29
Induction of labour			98
Care of the neonate			98
Handicapped neonates	40	23	97
Death of a baby			100
Family planning			78
Health promotion			45
b. Consent to treatment			
Informed consent	74	78	45
Patient autonomy	52	43	23
Patients' rights	52	63	
Patient protection	2	9	95
Maternal *vs* foetal rights			18
Confidentiality	51	86	78
Truth-telling	17	18	
Risk-taking	2★★	4★★	
c. Professionalism	64	74	
Code of Conduct			16
Accountability/Responsibility	48	56	88
Patient advocacy	68	56	
Quality assurance	19	21	
Interprofessional relationships	28	34	
Research ethics	2	8	46
d. Communication			56
Ethico-legal issues	35	45	
Religious/racial issues			12
Resources	15	33	

★ Courses in RMN training   ★★ Courses in Mental Handicap

Question 14
Are there any other topics/issues that you would like to deal with? If appropriate please indicate why these topics are not being covered at present.

68% of respondents felt that there were no essential topics that they were unable to deal with. However 54% said that shortage of staff and 78% said that shortage of time and the overcrowded curriculum prevented them dealing with all subjects in the detail they would wish.

12 tutors replied that they felt unable to handle some 'sensitive' issues although they were not very explicit about why they felt this way.

Question 15
What teaching methods are used for the study of ethics, e.g. lectures, discussions?

Teaching methods (%)	Type of Course						
	B	PB	C	M	M(C)	CE	UG
Formal lecture	25	18	6	20	16	45	84
Discussion	95	88	84	92	82	78	96
Debate	67	78	56	73	56	64	92
Role play	35	32	24	22	18	54	34
Project work	14	34	44	15	24	78	18

Question 16
Please specify which texts, videos or other teaching aids you find particularly useful.

Full details of the texts mentioned are contained in the bibliography. At this point it seems worth mentioning that tutors generally commented on the lack of suitable texts and teaching aids available to assist with the teaching of ethics. American texts, especially the case studies, are felt to be not entirely relevant, either organisationally, or legally.

Question 17
Is there some form of organisational structure or support system to help your staff cope with practical ethical problems?

28% responded that they felt a support structure did exist. Most of the 68% who replied in the negative did add that informal discussion with peers was usually found to be useful.

The hospital chaplain features heavily in most lists of support systems.

Support systems	% mentioned
Hospital chaplain	68
Peer group	73
Occupational Health	42
Senior Management	14
Counsellor	19
Ethical Committee	4
Health Authority	1

Appendix II

There are several special courses now available in the field of medical ethics, bioethics or philosophy of health care. These courses vary greatly in length, approach and content. The following list cannot be considered to provide a recommendation or to be exhaustive but merely a starting point for those interested.

Masters Degree

MA in Philosophy and Health Care Dr D Evans
Centre for the Study of Philosophy and Health Care
University College Swansea
Swansea
West Glamorgan

MA in Health Care Ethics
Dr J Harris
Dept of Philosophy
University of Manchester
Oxford Road
Manchester

MA in Medical Law and Ethics
Admissions Tutor
Centre for Law, Medicine and Ethics
Kings College
The Strand
London
W1

MA in Medical Ethics
Dr D Seedhouse
Dept of Medicine
University of Liverpool
Liverpool
Lancs

Masters Degrees are also believed to be in preparation in the universities of Hull and Leeds.

Shorter courses

Many short courses are now being developed in response to the growth of interest in ethics amongst practitioners. The above Universities often organise such events. Also

Dr R Gillon
Imperial College
Exhibition Road
London SW7

organises a short course in September of each year.

The Open University is always a useful resource especially for people who do not live near a college or university. It is in the middle of developing a module on ethics for the caring professions which it expects to have ready in late 1991.

Bibliography

Alexander M F (1983) Learning to Nurse. First Edition. Edinburgh: Churchill Livingstone.

Allen O H and Murrell J (1978) Nurse Training – an enterprise in curriculum development. First Edition. Plymouth: MacDonald and Evans.

Bergman R (1973) Ethics – Concepts and Practice. *International Nursing Review* Vol 20 September/October, pages 140–141, 152.

Blomquist C, Veatch R M and Fenner D (1975) The Teaching of Medical Ethics. *Journal of Medical Ethics*. Vol 1, Number 2: 96–103.

Branch M (1976) Models for introducing cultural diversity in Nursing curricula. *Journal of Nursing Education*. Vol 15: pages 7–13.

Brennan J M (1977) The Open-Texture of Moral Concepts. First Edition. London: The Macmillan Press Limited.

Brown S C (ed) (1975) Philosophers Discuss Education. First Edition. London: The Macmillan Press Limited.

Bunzl M (1975) A Note on Nursing Ethics in the U.S.A. *Journal of Medical Ethics*. Vol 1, Number 4: 184.

Button, L (1981) Group Tutoring for the Form Teacher. First Edition. London: Hodder and Stoughton.

Byerly E (1977) Cultural components in the baccalaureate nursing curriculum – philosophy, goals and processes. New York: National League for Nursing.

Campbell A V (1976) Moral Dilemmas in Medicine. Second Edition. Edinburgh: Churchill Livingstone.

Child D. (1981) Psychology and the Teacher. Third Edition. London: Holt, Rinehart and Winston.

Dickoff J and James P (1970) Beliefs and values: Bases for Curriculum design. *Nursing Research*. Vol 19, Number 5: 415–427.

Finnis J M (1980) Natural Law and Natural Rights. First Edition. Oxford: Oxford University Press.

Fletcher J (1967) Situation Ethics. First Edition. London: S.C.M. Press.

French P (1983) Social Skills for Nursing Practice. First Edition. London: Croom Helm.

Glover J (1984) Causing Death and Saving Lives. Sixth Edition. London: Penguin Books Limited.

Grazebrook J (1984) When the Chalking's Over. *Senior Nurse* Vol 1, Number 10: 30.

Hare R M (1963) Freedom and Reason. First Edition. Oxford: Oxford University Press.

Henderson V (1966) The Nature of Nursing. First Edition. London: Collier Macmillan.

Hirst P H (1975) Knowledge and the Curriculum: a collection of philosophical papers. First Edition. London: Routledge and Kegan Paul.

Hirst P H and Peters R S (1977) The logic of education. First Edition. London: Routledge and Kegan Paul.

Hoffman B (1962) The tyranny of testing. First Edition. New York: Cromwell Collier Press.

Johnson M (1983) Ethics in nurse education. *Nurse Education today*. Vol 3, Number 3: 58–59.

Kilbrandon Lord, Nuttal P D and Butrym Z (1975) Ethics and Professions. *Journal of Medical Ethics*. Vol 1, Number 1: 2–4.

Kohlberg L (1973) Continuities in childhood and adult word development revisited in *Life Span developmental psychology*. New York: Academic Press.

Kohlberg L (1978) The cognitive development approach in moral education in Scharf P (ed) *Readings in moral education*. Minneapolis: Winston Press.

Kramer M (1974) Reality Shock: Why nurses leave nursing. First Edition. St. Louis: C V Mosby Company.

Lancaster A (1980) Nursing and Midwifery Sourcebook. Second Edition. London: George Allen and Unwin.

Leininger M (1978) Cultural and Transcultural nursing. New York: National League for Nursing.

Lello J (1979) Accountability in Education. First Edition. London: Ward Lock Educational.

Loukes H (1957) Progress and Problems in Moral Education. First Edition. Slough: National Foundation for Educational Research.

McPhail P (1982) Social and Moral Education. First Edition. Oxford: Blackwell Publishers Limited.

Moore G E (1966) *Ethics*. First Edition. Oxford: Oxford University Press.

Norman R (ed) (1975) The Neutral Teacher, in Brown C S: Philosophers discuss education. First Edition. London: The Macmillan Press Limited.

Oakeshott M (1975) On Human Conduct. First Edition. London: Oxford University Press.

Paton H J (1969) The Moral Law: Kants Groundwork of the Metaphysics of Morals. First Edition. London: Hutchinson University Library.

Peters R S (1979) Authority, responsibility and education. Fifth Edition. Boston: George Allen and Unwin.

Piaget J. (1965) The moral judgment of the child. Second Edition. New York: Free Press.

Rabb J D (1976) Implications of moral and ethical issues for nurses. *Nursing Forum*. Vol 15, Number 2: 168–179.

Rensburg P van (1974) Report from Swaneng Hill. London: The Dag Hammarskjold Foundation.

Rodmell F E (1985) Moral Education – a review of the curriculum input. Unpublished paper.

Ross D (1969) Kants Ethical Theory. First Edition. Oxford: Oxford University Press.

Swider S M, McElmurry B J and Yarling R R (1985) Ethical decision-making in a bureaucratic context by senior nursing students. *Nursing Research*. Vol 34, Number 2: 108–112.

Toulmin S (1958) The Place of Reason in Ethics. First Edition. Cambridge: Cambridge University Press.

Turner C (1985) Patient Education. *Senior Nurse*. Vol 2, Number 2: 10–12.

Warnock M (1975) The Neutral Teacher, in Brown C S (ed) Philosophers discuss Education. First Edition. London: The Macmillan Press Limited.

Watt A J (1976) Rational Moral Education. First Edition. Melbourne: Melbourne University Press.

Weidenback E (1970) Comment on: Beliefs and values: Bases for Curriculum design. *Nursing Research*. Vol 19, Number 5: 427.

Further Reading

Basic Texts

A) Ethical theory

Beauchamp Tom L (1982) Philosophical Ethics: An Introduction to Moral Philosophy. New York: McGraw Hill.

Brandt Richard B (1979) A Theory of the Good and Right. Oxford: Clarendon Press.

Frankena William K (1973). Ethics. 2nd Edition Englewood Cliffs, N.J.: Prentice Hall.

Hare R M. (1981) Moral Thinking: Its Levels, Methods and Point. Oxford: Clarendon Press.

Rawls John (1971) A Theory of Justice. Cambridge, Mass.: Harvard University Press.

Singer Peter (1979) Practical Ethics. Cambridge: Cambridge University Press.

B) Biomedical ethics

Beauchamp Tom L and Childress James F (1989) Principles of Biomedical Ethics. 3rd Edition. New York: Oxford University Press.

Brody Howard (1981) Ethical decisions in Medicine. 2nd Edition. Boston: Little, Brown and Company.

Campbell Alastair V (1975) Moral Dilemmas in Medicine. 2nd Edition. Edinburgh: Churchill Livingston.

Childress James F (1981) Priorities in Biomedical Ethics. Philadelphia: The Westminster Press.

Glover Jonathan (1977) Causing Death and Saving Lives. New York: Penguin Books.

McCormick Richard A (1981) How Brave New World? Dilemmas in Bioethics. Garden City, N.Y.: Doubleday.

Ramsey Paul (1978) Ethics at the Edge of Life. New Haven: Yale University Press.

Veatch Robert M (1981) A Theory of Medical Ethics. New York: Basic Books, Inc.

C) Nursing texts

Baly M. (1984) Professional Responsibility. 2nd Edition. Chichester: John Wiley and Sons.

Benjamin M and Curtis J (1981) Ethics in Nursing. New York: Oxford University Press.

Brykczynska Gosia M (1989) Ethics in Paediatric Nursing. London: Chapman and Hall.

Curtin L and Flaherty M J (1982) Nursing Ethics: Theories and Pragmatics. Englewood Cliffs, N.J.: Prentice Hall International Inc.

Davis A J and Aroskar M A (1983) Ethical Dilemmas and Nursing Practice. Norwalk, Conn.: Appleton-Century-Crofts.

Fletcher J (1967) Moral Responsibility: Situation Ethics at Work. London: SCM Press.

Jameton A (1984) Nursing Practice: the Ethical Issues. Englewood Cliffs, N.J.: Prentice Hall.

Mayeroff M (1972) On Caring. New York: Harper and Row.

Steele S M and Harmon V M (1983) Values Clarification in Nursing 2nd Edition. Norwalk, Conn.: Appleton-Century-Crofts.

Thompson I A, Melia K and Boyd K (1989) Nursing Ethics. Edinburgh: Churchill Livingstone.

Tschudin Verena (1986) Ethics in Nursing: the caring relationship. London: Heinemann.

Veatch Robert M and Fry Sarah T (1987) Case Studies in Nursing Ethics. Philadelphia: J B Lipincott.

References

Goldman S A and Arbuthnot J (1979) *Teaching Medical Ethics: The Cognitive–Development Approach. Journal of Medical Ethics*, **5**: 170–181.

Murdock I (1985) *The Sovereignty of Good*. London: Ark Paperbacks.

Royal College of Nursing (1977) RCN Code of Professional Conduct: a discussion document. *Journal of Medical Ethics*, **3**: 115–123.

Royal College of Nursing (1980) *Guidelines on Confidentiality in Nursing*. London: RCN.

United Kingdom Central Council for Nursing, Midwifery and Health Visiting (1984) *Code of Professional Conduct for the Nurse, Midwife and Health Visitor*, 2nd ed. London: UKCC.

United Kingdom Central Council for Nursing, Midwifery and Health Visiting, Educational Policy Advisory Committee (1985) *Project 2000: Project Papers 1–4*. London: UKCC.

Yura H and Walsh M B (1978) *The Nursing Process: Assessing, Planning, Implementing, Evaluating*, 3rd ed. New York: Appleton-Century-Crofts.